Motivated to Inspire

A cancer survivor's perspective

Alfred Samuels

The Cloister House Press

First published in the United Kingdom in 2017
by The Cloister House Press
ISBN 978-1909465572

Contents

For all cancer survivors: you can do the things you think

you cannot do – your life is not over, it's just starting

Dedications & acknowledgements

First and foremost, I would like to thank my wife, Grace, for standing beside me throughout my serious illness. She has been my inspiration and motivation for continuing to live. She is my rock, and I dedicate this book to her. I also thank my wonderful children, who are just about the best children a dad could want. You have always made me smile during the days, weeks and months when I was writing this book instead of spending quality time with you. I hope that one day you can read this book and understand why I spent so much time in front of my computer.

I am not nearly so strong as I imagine myself to be. 'But by the grace of God I am what I am, and his grace toward me was not in vain.' (1 Cor. 15:3)

The late Gordon Holt – never a truer dear friend. R.I.P.

Pete Axson (a prostate cancer warrior and brother). Thank you for inspiring me further.

The doctors and nurses of the Oncology Department, Mount Vernon Cancer Treatment Centre, Mount Vernon Hospital, Hertfordshire, UK.

Cancer Research UK

Preface: Why I wrote this book

The answer is actually quite simple. I have a great deal of experience in the area of prostate cancer from a survivor's perspective and, therefore, something worthwhile to talk about. We all have varying experiences in life, from junior school to high school and maybe even university. We have experiences in relationships with girlfriends and boyfriends. We also have experiences with people in general, through work or as neighbours. Everyone has a unique story to tell; mine is about my journey and perspective with prostate cancer and it is my desire to share it with the world. This is the result of that work and my continuing story.

When preparing to write this book I read a great deal online, not only about prostate cancer but about cancer in general. Much of the information was complicated. Instead of taking the time to describe how all the pieces fit together, everyone seemed more interested in writing complex physician jargon that caused the lay person to nod, twist and jerk in agony about something that should be quite simple to understand. What was missing from all of the publications was the understandable version, which I hope I am able to describe. I decided this was how I wanted to address my book.

Lastly, I wrote this book because I'm passionate about the topic of cancer and what organisations like Cancer Research UK are doing. I sincerely believe there will be a cure in the not-too-distant future.

Over the last decade, a fundamental change has occurred in the way the medical world and big pharmaceuticals have approached cancer and its treatment. There are numerous advances in oncology treatments to be excited about – from immunotherapy to vaccines and monoclonal antibodies – but unfortunately, cancer is such a complex disease that none of these are guaranteed to work for every patient.

However, on the horizon sits 'precision medicine', which may be the answer. Also known as personalised medicine, it involves giving patients the best treatments based on specific genetic biomarkers. Through advanced diagnostic tests, precise differences in patients' genes can be taken into account when examining their illness, and then a drug that suits these factors can be prescribed. This excites me and many other cancer survivors, researchers, and academics. It sounds, and is, simple, but it is a genuine departure from standard treatments like chemotherapy, whose one-size-fits-all approach can be successful for some patients but not others. Clinical trials are critical in developing new treatments and better understanding the biology of the disease. As a patient who has enrolled in such trials, namely the STAMPEDE programme, I have had the advantage of being among the first to receive the newest drugs and drug combinations. I received close scrutiny and monitoring on my trials programme and can attest to its value. In my opinion, the more people who enrol, the faster researchers will be able to find answers.

I truly believe that, once you get a glimpse of the bigger picture, you'll change the way you look at the overall outcome and with your viewpoint changed, your survivability is realistic.

Alfred Samuels

1: My story

During October 2011, I was in a London hospital A&E room with severe lower back pain that radiated down my right leg. A few months later it turned out I had a previously undiagnosed widespread metastatic prostate cancer disease. Fast-tracked straight to my regional hospital oncology department, I soon commenced treatment under the 'STAMPEDE' (Systemic Therapy in Advancing or Metastatic Prostate Cancer: Evaluation of Drug Efficacy) trials programme at age 54.

'STAMPEDE is a randomised controlled trial using a multi-arm, multi-stage platform design. It recruits men with high-risk, locally advanced, metastatic or recurrent prostate cancer who are starting first-line long-term hormone therapy. The aim of this trial is to try to prevent the tumour re-growth by adding other treatment to the hormone therapy. The trial is currently assessing abiraterone and enzalutamide in combination with hormone therapy or radiotherapy (newly diagnosed metastatic patients only) in combination with hormone therapy.' *(www.stampedetrial.org/)*

I am currently living with advanced metastatic prostate cancer, and I am certainly not waiting to die from it. That said, I am also very aware as an optimistic realist that while treatment is helpful, and still allows a reasonable quality of life, then I choose life. The alternative is not one I wish to embrace too early and without reason and, until my last breath, I will hold peace, hope, and love in my heart. I understand, and indeed am thankful that for now, I have time to plan, experience life, make memories with those around me and I hope to continue to do so for a long time yet. Many do not get that chance as their time comes swiftly and without warning. I have watched too many friends pass from this disease and it is not 'best' in any way.

Cancer treatment is NEVER fun or easy, and it is an educated guess as to whether each treatment will help or hinder your overall health, or indeed, not impact on your cancer at all and, just because we may look good on the outside, it rarely matches what's inside. I just work on having as many good days as possible and work harder to get through the not-so-good ones. I wish it was just that simple. Sort yourself out, and then off for an easy and peaceful passing. Oh, and that would be while not needing to constantly swallow a major drug factory or being injected to keep you 'comfortable'. Life is just not that simple, and when the time comes to embrace death, it is still not simple.

Advancements in treatments have given us, on average, more time than in the past but it is still a difficult, trying and exhausting path where the best we can do is be happy if we gain a good test or report, hear the words 'stable' or 'no evidence of disease' and, in the meantime, live life every single day, keep smiling, deal with each treatments side effects or progression as it happens and just keep on putting one foot in front of the other.

For the last five years of my life, I have struggled with this disease and I have now reached that milestone and the magic number: five years post-diagnosis. In doing so, I am entering the last phase of a three-pronged journey: Living with cancer; living through cancer, living beyond cancer.

My mind, body, and soul have been subjected to physical and emotional horror through these stages, and at times relief can seem to be an unbearably long way off.

When I was first diagnosed, while I was in the stage of living with cancer, I never for one instant thought I would make it. This is the treatment stage where it all starts: surgery, chemotherapy, and radiation. Depending on how far your cancer has progressed, the treatment may accelerate, which means in other words that surgery may not be an option, so chemo via intravenous (IV) or tablets is the first possible course of action. In my opinion, living with cancer is one of the hardest stages. Consulting regularly with your doctor becomes the norm.

The next stage is living through cancer. This is the stage after treatment, better known as the transition phase. It is during this stage that many so-called survivors struggle with finding their 'new normal'. Some may feel that their cancer has changed them: their perspective, their personality, their lifestyle. Many are afraid that their cancer will make a comeback.

Survivors see their consultant less often than they did in the previous stage, to have what is known as 'active surveillance care' carried out.

Last, but not least, is the living beyond cancer stage. This lasts for years after cancer treatment: you may find yourself living beyond cancer. You enter the long-term survival stage. You start to find that the feeling of normality within you is returning. By now you have learnt to deal with the remnants of the fight in your daily life. Appointments with your oncologist are now becoming less frequent as your care is handed over to your family doctor.

It is very important to look forward always, regardless of the stage. It does not matter whether you see yourself as a fighter, warrior, or survivor: you may even reject all of these labels. It's a personal choice. The 'new normal' is where you are at: now you have to try to make it work. No matter what you do, remembering to continue to fight, something which, by now, you are certainly an expert at.

When one lives in a state of near-permanent pain, it brings about all sorts of mixed mental emotions. Accepting that some things in life cannot be fixed is far removed from 'they can only be carried', but ultimately this is the reality of the situation. Many of us do not accept, and we live in the world of advice, in denial and unable to accept this turmoil. However, those of us who do accept, generally find the one thing we must do as our lives are turned upside down: grieve.

Grief is brutal and undeniably painful. Grief does not only occur when someone dies. For example, when relationships fall apart you grieve. When illness ravages you, you grieve. Being diagnosed with a debilitating illness cannot be fixed. This can only be carried. Yes, devastation can lead to growth, but it often doesn't. It often destroys lives – in part because we've replaced grieving with advice. With platitudes. For me, I now live an extraordinary life. I've been deeply blessed by the opportunities I've had and the radically unconventional life that I've built for myself – this I call 'a new beginning'. Above all, I've been left with a pervasive survivor's guilt that has haunted me for the past five years. In short, my pain has never gone away – I've just learned to channel it into my work with others. Discussing with family is very difficult – we don't normally talk about our feelings, neither do family. But we all know it's there. We are private about it and have our own little moments where we cry. We don't do it together often – I don't think I'm scared of actually dying, just the lead up to that exit point. Seeing people for the last time; I just cannot imagine it.

I am by no means encompassing everyone: just remember there are different stories and experiences for each and every one of us undergoing this journey.

Connecting with other cancer patients, caregivers and loved ones in person is quite a great source of support, strength and encouragement for people living with cancer. Sharing your experiences with others can help you in not only accepting your condition but also in feeling comfortable that you are not alone in your struggle with this disease and that there is a light at the end of the so-called tunnel. Cancer leaves you with an overwhelming feeling of uncertainty about what lies ahead as you travel through the very unfamiliar world of cancer. When you network you will meet like-minded people most of whom are in treatment or post-treatment phases. From those people you will learn what the journey ahead consists of and looks like, which will help to dampen the fears and anxieties you are undergoing.

From a personal perspective, trying to go through cancer alone is not advisable. It will torture you by tearing you apart far more slowly and the pain of that is unimaginable for sure. Clearly, you will have questions resting on your mind, some of which could be: How do I keep up with the tasks of everyday living? Who do I ask for support? If you have not already done so: How do I inform my family and close friends as to my plight and how can they assist me? It is very important that those around you are there to help, and not burden you, as can so often happen.

It is easier said than done to have a supportive care team around you. It takes careful planning and coordination so that those involved do not burden you or burn out or overwhelm you in a bid to assist you. If managed correctly, it keeps the patient from seeming to be asking for the assistance that they need, which can be humiliating at times, I can tell you. Organisations such as Cancer Research UK and Macmillan are among a few that provide a bona fide source of networking support for cancer patients.

2: A day in my life, fighting for my tomorrow

Many mornings when I rise, I feel that I have been sledge-hammered into a pulp. As I lay horizontal, burbling out words that are unintelligible, I try to focus on a new day. The new day: more medication, finding more resolve to deal with the shit I am going through with this cancer journey. Another day of dealing with a society that lacks a real understanding of the complexities of that whose only role is to destroy me and end my life.

There are those days I rise full of vigour clenching my fists like a trained boxer, feeling the power that exists within my body to force out and dissipate the energy of a powerful nature sufficient to cause a knockout punch. Clearly, these are far and few between moments. 'The mind is strong, but the body is weak' is a cliché that befalls me for most of my days.

Clear, concise thoughts evade me most days as I struggle with brain fog, just another side effect I have to encounter in a bid to remain consciously awake and functional. You may wonder why I would wish to remain alive under such circumstances, and you would be correct in this thinking.

I have to remain driven and focused, because the desire to think negatively arrives in a flash. Before me, a host of people – wife, children, siblings, friends – all wishing me well, all rooting for me for all that I do to rise above my daily dance with this disease. The love, the admiration, the support, the intrinsic value – when combined they all should bring a cure in itself for any ailment faced. Sadly, in reality, this is not the case. From within our shell, we look out into the wide world through eyes that show and speak suffering.

How do I communicate to people the numbness that graces my daily thought process? I sit writing, struggling to find a structure to sentences that before this disease would have come easily. I am alive: I know this because I pinch myself every day and feel the pain of the nip, but I am still stuck in my mind and body trying to reach out and make others understand what ails me and how it affects me.

On many occasions I have conversed with my wife as we talk through the material for my writing, knowing what I want to say but finding those impactful words elusive, sometimes arrogantly suggesting that a group of words would suffice until I had time to decipher my thought at a later date. This is the 'me' that now exists; this is the 'me' that struggles to co-exist in a far more complex world than that of many years ago. We live in a world now ruled by this evolving technology – which the kids of today have grown up around – placing great pressure on adults to keep pace. As technology and the human race advance, I fight in my headspace to break free from this deadlock. In the blink of an eye, my life changed, and I was not ready for it. I am sure that if I were granted the opportunity for a rewind, it would not make an ounce of difference to today's outcome because that's what the blink of an eye does.

From here on, your dreams, goals, and priorities are forced to take different turns, but sometimes some of these are into cul-de-sacs and the complexity of that turn becomes too much to deal with. This is now your life, and only you can deal with its dramas as you cannot make others understand what you are going through because the condition dictates otherwise. Even now I am wondering if I am coming across to my reading audience clearly. Am I getting through to you to how clouded, muddled, and disengaged this condition has made me? Those who do understand are few and far between, and most of these I have found in online forums where stories are posted. It is here that one finds understanding and logic in my world of cancer.

Right now, my quality of life and bone health has been maintained. Most mornings now when I rise, I mutter a little perk-me-up to myself: 'Not much time to think about possibilities; there's no reason to worry. The Lord is in control. I know that He still has much work for me to do and I believe He has given me this time to help others with raising awareness of this lethal cancer that tries to steal life, laughter, and love from its next target.'

The mortality statistics show there are 36 prostate cancer deaths for every 100,000 males in the UK. I have remained one of those who has not fallen into these statistics. Each month, however, a grey cloud hovers above me, because you just don't know what the outcome will be at the next PSA test.

Accompanying me at most of these hospital result sessions is my wife, Grace. She sits on the edge, pondering the possibilities of her loved one, not realising that I, myself, am on tenterhooks. The one thing that has come out of all of this is that our family has become closer, stronger, and is prepared for whatever news happens to me. There is a realisation – having witnessed the demise of my mother, her sister and her brother – that this family may need to prepare themselves to fight the cancer fight for generations to come.

I have learnt many lessons from my cancer journey. Fighting prostate cancer remains the hardest thing I've done in my life. Being in the hospital with other patients, some of whom knew they wouldn't win their battle, I came to see that peace is always there. No matter the circumstances, no matter the ugliness of the challenge before me, giving up was not an option. After a few months of my cancer journey, I decided I didn't want my fight to include a lack of communication between myself and my immediate family. I'd seen other people fight cancer, and I always felt that there was a certain amount of silence to it. It felt like we were all scared to say or ask certain questions or raise points. I didn't want my fight to be like that. I wanted to talk openly about what I was experiencing, and I wanted to ask very important questions along the way. The important questions were always worth asking, even when the answer wasn't a happy one.

From herein, my life's work is to share what I have learned so that it can help other men, including cancer survivors, to live happier, healthier, more fulfilling lives. I continue to do this through my writings.

3: The infinite resilience of the human spirit

I never realised the resilience within me would carry me through my cancer journey into the present day. I suppose there were a number of things that I implemented unknowingly, to ensure that this resilience was permanent. My daily routine from dawn to dusk was all about cancer, from medication to treatment appointments, to discussing daily with my partner and family about the disease. There was never a let-up about this disease in my daily life until I started to do things outside of cancer and incorporated them into my daily routine thereafter.

Hill walking with a weighted backpack pushed me beyond my usual physical boundaries. Mentoring children at state schools gave me an absolute buzz of self-appreciation. These were just a few of the things I became involved with and, as such, my secluded home affair became a thing of the past as I ventured more out into the wide world. My mind had at long last found new and meaningful things to attach itself to.

To complement the stresses and worries, I was facing financial hardship, family discontent and intimacy issues that were paralysing my life. The financial losses were the hardest to overcome. I watched as everything I had worked for in life started to fall apart around me. I had invested heavily into a major business venture that was yet to bear fruit. I could not claw back these funds, so I walked that long, dark, empty tunnel of financial ruin: if only I could claw those funds back, how my life would be turned around. Long-term investments are what they say– long-term; you invest your money and take your chances.

Though I was the person diagnosed, this was not the only case to consider. Whilst it was clear that cancer was rife in the family, my mind was flipping over and over that the prostate cancer that I was facing could also be faced by my sons at a later date. This only added a deeper sense of concern for my family, and bringing about a sense of calm and nullifying scaremongering was my priority. An open dialogue was something I entered into with my sons and my younger brother, and I insisted on a sense of active surveillance so that the message was clear as they walked through life: take nothing for granted.

There then came the most sensitive and emotional issue, that of intimacy, which I at first closed my eyes and heart to simply because I could not manage. This was so heartbreaking, as I enjoyed such a passionate relationship with my partner prior to my diagnosis. Now here I was struggling to be intimate, passionate and loving to the woman who had cared for me and subsequently saved my life. My love for my partner was undeniable, but to find yourself stripped of the feelings that once existed was insurmountable.

Giving our relationship much thought, however, it became clear that we were friends before lovers and, for later, this is even stronger than at the beginning. I am only stripped of that which suggests that intimacy to many means the intimacy of intercourse, without which you have nothing. The news is that ours is not that and does not rest on that, since we have meticulously taken care of every little thing, to make the whole experience of loving one another a truly memorable one away from intercourse alone.

My days prior to my diagnosis never allowed for a moment of let-up in my hectic lifestyle. There was never a moment to reflect or ease the pressure on my mind as I battled in the mean business world of making money. The Spanish have it down to a tee – siesta. It's amazing the difference one or two hours of rest midday makes on the mind and body.

Here I was attempting to withstand the worst illness of my life with a view to bouncing back. I was not going to allow myself to stay broken as the illness would have had me do. Working hard to overcome my situation became my blossoming inner strength. Though I do suspect that it was and is always there, I just had to reach deep down inside to find it. The mirror and 1 became very good friends indeed, as on a daily basis I sought clarification as to why this had happened to me. I sought to watch my body's physical shape change into something of a monstrosity as my steroid medication increased my waistline, swelling my body into that of a beer- guzzling, burger eating male.

One thing about the mirror: it never lied to me. It reflected the true situation and circumstances that stood before it, and that was hard to accept as each day I groaned at what I was seeing. But I stayed strong until I started to see the transcendence in the mirror and I began to love 'me' again. This chaotic mess before the mirror had somehow managed to organise the chaos into a reasonably stable and person of worth again. And as Carl Jung understood, 'our ego must deal not only with extended challenges but also challenges from archetypal psychic energies which press from the inside demanding expression in our individual lives.'

My resilience to the extreme situation that I was facing did not allow me to put into place or develop an all-option mechanism. How was I to withstand this outrageous attack on my body, this criminal, life-limiting, brutal invasion of my form? We live in an orderly world and the impact on my life led me to question my faith with the Almighty. Why me? As I looked deeper into me, the answers started to become clearer from the reflective instrument before me.

I'm not the first to be diagnosed with cancer; children and adults alike live through traumatic experiences with their spirit relatively intact. I am fortunately one of those, but I do feel for those who are left permanently damaged by the diagnosis. What is it that makes me or people like me different from them? Have they lived a bad life and this was their punishment, a reflection of something in their personality makeup or some genetic component of their character? Trying to disassociate myself from their unbearable trauma proved far harder than I had imagined; trying to create an internal physical barricade against this indigestible shocking experience was to prove the challenge of challenges.

In my case, the sudden, dramatic change that occurred through being diagnosed proved to be unquestionably the pivotal point in my life.

4: Cancer and the importance of networking

One thing is for sure: I'm getting older and finding that I hurt more often than not. I creak more, and at times I shuffle around the home instead of taking the bounding strides I once took. Of course, another grey hair appears on my chin for my wife and her tweezers to pull out, and I now need all of my eight to ten hours' sleep. But I am alive, and the aforementioned is a luxury considering the dire circumstances that I faced in January 2012 as an advanced metastatic prostate cancer diagnosis put my life at a standstill.

Compelling matters was that I came from a family of cancer fatalities, as I watched my mother, my aunt and my uncle all lose their battle against cancer.

Today cancer is the biggest disease on the cultural map, bigger even than cystic fibrosis, AIDS or spinal injury. Bigger even than the five prolific killers of men – strokes, liver disease, coronary heart disease and respiratory diseases (the two main ones being asthma and chronic obstructive pulmonary disease or COPD). There are numerous websites that are devoted to it all, not to mention newsletters, support groups and a whole new genre of prostate cancer books.

As I waded into the relevant online cancer support groups, the first thing I discovered was that not everyone views the disease with a negative emotional reaction. Instead, you meet upbeat attitudes and even a somewhat avaricious craving for more knowledge about the disease at hand. There is no doubt, though, that the intention of these websites is to inspire a positive outlook, regardless of the grading or Gleason score.

I needed whatever help I could get and eventually found myself searching fanatically for answers to my own dilemma and, surprisingly, found some very good answers in these forums. But, for me personally, nothing was better than my one-to-one conversations with my own oncologist. There is, I found, a significant market for all these chat rooms, although better moderation is required. You can't have someone coming online and claiming to be an oncologist, giving out advice to people: how do we know whether they are who they say they are? Most importantly, every cancer sufferer goes through and deals with cancer differently, so the one-to-one interaction will always be paramount to a sufferer.

Connecting with other cancer patients, caregivers and loved ones in person is a great source of support, strength, and encouragement for people dealing with cancer. Sharing your experiences with others can help you in not only accepting your condition but also in feeling comfortable that you are not alone in your struggle with this disease and that there is light at the end of the so-called tunnel. Cancer leaves you with an overwhelming feeling of uncertainty about what lies ahead as you travel through this very unfamiliar new world.

When you network you will meet like-minded people, most of whom are undergoing treatment or are in post-treatment phases. From those people, you will learn what the journey ahead consists of and looks like, which will help to dampen the fears and anxieties you are undergoing. From a personal perspective, trying to go through cancer alone is not advisable. It will torture you by tearing you apart far more slowly, and that pain is unimaginable for sure. Clearly, you will have questions resting on your mind, some of which could be – How do I keep up with the tasks of everyday living? Who do I ask for support from? If you have not already done so – How do I inform my family and close friends about my plight and how can they assist me? It is very important that those around you are there to help and not burden you, as can so often happen.

To have a supportive care team around you is easier said than done. It takes careful planning and coordination such that persons involved do not burden you or burn out or overwhelm you in a bid to assist you. If managed correctly, it keeps the patient from seeming to be asking for the assistance that they need, which can be a humiliating feeling at times, I can tell you.

Organisations such as Cancer Research UK, Macmillan, and Prostate Cancer UK are amongst a few that provide a bona fide source of networking support and service for cancer patients.

In the mainstream of cancer culture, there is very little anger, no mention of possible environmental causes, and few comments about the fact that, in all but the more advanced metastasised cases, it is the 'treatments', not the disease, that cause the immediate illness and pain. In fact, the overall tone is almost universally upbeat.

When one takes, for example, the 'Breast Friends' website, which features a series of inspirational quotes – 'Don't cry over anything that can't cry over you'; 'When life hands out lemons, squeeze out a smile'; 'Don't wait for your ship to come in: swim out to meet it,' and many more of that ilk – it can be seen that cancer, on the whole, has moved on from 'the grim reaper is coming for you' to this universally upbeat tone of survival.

In the midst of this hell, I have also somehow found the strength to live as a survivor and not as a cancer patient because the two, in my mind, are intrinsically very different. There is the school of thought that suggests some people who have been diagnosed with cancer reject the term 'survivor' or disagree with some definitions of it. Personally speaking, I believe it boils down to the individual undergoing the journey as to where they see themselves, and nobody else, because this is their journey and no one can walk it but them.

As humans, we tend to think that a diagnosis of this magnitude would tear us apart, but when you look back and reflect on your journey, you can see just how much it has inspired and built you up, especially when surrounded with the new network around you. It's a wondrous thing when we can inspire ourselves, and how our strengths and journeys can subsequently inspire others.

I wanted so desperately to pick up where I left off. I couldn't help but feel like I had to go back where it all began. But God put me in a much better place. I am so thankful for my fight because it has made me the man that I am today. Without my fight, I wouldn't know this amazing new man who is so full of zest and life and his new-found circle.

5: Thoughts, behaviours and emotions during cancer

The statistics suggest that one in three cancer patients suffers from mental health issues. I am a survivor of the disease and as such have found myself grappling with its tentacles. The thing that almost broke me, though, was the torturous mental aspect of my situation. I found that the battle in my mind was actually harder than the battle in my body.

You have to try and see it from my perspective. Prior to being diagnosed with, in my case, prostate cancer, I was in the best shape of my life and everything was going so well. Then along came the diagnosis and it broke my spirit for a while. I lost all my bodily hair, I lost weight and became a monster of a person and on many occasions mentally I was not myself. My mind and body were subjected to an onslaught of continuous invasive treatment.

Everybody who has gone through any kind of chemotherapy treatment knows about the moments when you say to yourself, I can't do this anymore, I want to give up. From the onset of treatment, there is fundamental trust in one's body that says: you will get through this ordeal. As the treatment is introduced and fed into your organs, that feeling changes and becomes a feeling of, I don't have energy or inclination like I used to have to continue. Isolation will creep into your every day; feeling socially isolated as a cancer patient is a submissive and awful feeling. It becomes clear sooner rather than later that you can't do this journey by yourself, therefore, reverting to therapy treatment is highly recommended because, in reality, you need someone professional and of a non-kin persuasion. Feeling that you're not alone aids in the mental health process of getting through this journey and when combined with the social support it can help to reduce cancer-related depression.

Like a true warrior I tried my utmost to remain strong, as I stood up to cancer, subconsciously always saying to myself that I was not going to let it take me from myself and loved ones, but like most things in life this was not to be an easy task at all. Physically I was strong but mentally I was not prepared and I bordered on the verge of giving up.

Being diagnosed with cancer and undergoing treatment can impact upon a patient's mental well-being. A cancer diagnosis is a life-changing event. It can be overwhelming to deal with cancer treatment and its side effects, while also handling the normal stresses of everyday life. To deal with any diagnosis of cancer makes one dig deep into your subconscious where you find the mental strength to cope and continue. For me, developing the mental strength to cope with this diagnosis was a three-pronged approach. It was about controlling my thoughts, behaviours and emotions, of which each takes not just a nibble but a chunk out of you.

At a recent Christmas gathering amongst friends, the question was raised to me about my mental state throughout my cancer journey.

I recalled saying that at any moment during my day a sudden, word, picture or thought might place me back into my subconscious and for a moment I am thrown back into the melee of it all again.

Unlike the early days of my journey, when I did not know how to control my thoughts, I was now a master of this aspect; at least I thought I was. Anger about why I was burdened with this awful disease no longer plays on my mind; you see, I have accepted it. It had to be someone, so why not me? Of course, the emotional turmoil forced itself on me and mine, but together we as a family fought it.

The frequent hormone injections tore at my emotional strings and, for me, this was the hardest to win over because it was a drug medically induced into my system, where no family or friends can go and help or partake, unlike the other approaches. Communicating the sad and difficult news to my children and siblings was by far the worst thing I have ever had to do in my life. It set me up for being able to keep my emotions under control when having to talk to people in general about my disease. Little did I realise that I would, in years to come, talk to audiences in the thousands or be watched by millions on a TV network.

Keeping it all in was possibly the biggest mistake that I made. The 'iron man' mentality does not work, as it will get you eventually. My change came about without warning; as Christmas 2015 approached I began to feel somewhat withdrawn and more concerned about my condition than at any time previously. I found that I did not want to share this feeling with my partner nor male family members. The days became weeks and this feeling continued. Then the occasion arose to make an 'I bring you tidings of joy' visit to my oncologist, and I planned to surprise him with a homemade Christmas cake.

When the day came, and I entered his office, I recall that he immediately realised something was wrong, and I tried to hide it without success. Once I had handed over the cake, my eyes welled up and the tears followed closely. I was asked to sit, and for the next thirty minutes a conversation took place between us. I found that I poured out all that had been bothering and saddening me. The strategy of the three-pronged approach was missing something. I had experienced mood changes, leading to the need to talk with someone professionally about what was concerning me.

'No man is an island,' as my father had always said, and here I was trying to be just that – an island. In reality, though, I was well, my cancer was under control and my prostate-specific antigen (PSA) had not budged over 0.1 for three years. In the words of my oncologist: you are a miracle case.

6: *That small voice*

Since the beginning of time, humans have talked about a 'small voice' that speaks to us from the core of our being in moments of danger or great intensity and direct us to safety or towards our destiny.

It has often been interpreted as the soul or the voice of God. Personally, I believe that what I am hearing is the voice of my inner wisdom, of my consciousness, the sum of memory and all my experiences, which takes over my internal dialogue regardless of the type of cancer and whether it is at an early or late stage.

I have advanced metastatic prostate cancer, but as I have said many times before, prostate cancer does not have me. Two choices were placed in front of me: give up or fight. Knowing that the disease was an aggressive type put me in a frame of mind that I too was going to be aggressive in dealing with it. The fact is that cancer turns your life upside down and inside out. I am now 58, and I have lived a fruitful life full of excitement and travel. Should my number be called tomorrow, I am ready for that spiritual departure from this world to wherever it takes me next. On many occasions, my thoughts took me in different directions, nothing more than that of the plight of youngsters who are experiencing cancer. The same can't be said about their lives, which have really only just begun.

They have so much of their life yet to live, and hopes and dreams to achieve. No matter what age you are, when a cancer diagnosis is given, it casts a dark cloud over your life. For those of a younger age, it is a difficult adjustment to make at a time when you're supposed to be brimming with optimism about your future. I suppose the same could be said of someone of my age, someone who should now be looking forward, too, and not facing a life-threatening, energy-sapping illness. 'Was it all really worth it?' I often ask myself.

My feelings are invisible, and I understand this because it is the same process of ignoring the pain that led me to this avenue. There are times that I feel so low that I become good at hiding it even from myself as I struggle daily. As each day passes, the mask that I wear sits more firmly on my face, protecting me and those I love as I continue to hold on. You see, it's hard to keep living when your life feels as if it has stopped. I can't do all the things that I used to do when I was whole. I can't just get up and move around like before. I can't help around the kitchen like I used to. I have to think about every move I make and the crucial impact that it can have. Whether that is walking down the road, going to a meeting, going shopping, exercising, everything: I get tearful at times when my mind rests on some or all of these issues. All that is happening inside me is invisible to those around me, as the mask continues to shield. As I think, I also talk to myself internally.

Today my PSA is undetectable. The regular check-ups continue, and I am in love with a wonderful woman who keeps me moving forward. Even though I try to hide much from her, she sees through the mask.

Without her, many of the medical terms used to describe my condition by my medical team would have flown over my head. Everyone who sees me now would never know that I have metastatic prostate cancer. Nobody would know. I owe all of this to my wife. She takes care of me. I tell people this all the time. I could never have done this by myself: she is my rock. She attended the majority of my appointments with me. She does not attend many now because I am doing so well, but she's always there in spirit, even texting me questions to ask my oncologist. She's my advocate. She explains medical terms that I don't understand and asks the questions I don't know how to ask. She has always been there for me.

Still, I exist: the living is on hold. I want to be open and honest about my experience, but it is a very hard thing to do. It is scary for me to show others what is beneath the mask I wear.

I share this in the hope that you, the reader, do not think I ask for pity or sympathy, because I do not. No one knows the pain, distress, or whatever you want to name it that a cancer survivor goes through. I am just trying for myself to be seen in my vulnerable state in a written format rather than some video on YouTube – after all, that's what those who wear masks do. I suppose I just want people to listen rather than converse because in most instances they are only going to say the wrong things. I just want to help and inspire other men.

Nowadays my upbeat manner and outlook help other men as they find their way back from the diagnosis of prostate cancer and through treatment and recovery. I am often on a soapbox telling men to get checked, because what really worries me is that men who aren't getting checked sometimes find out they have prostate cancer when it's too late, like I did. That bothers me a great deal. Men's biggest problem is talking about prostate cancer, the fear of losing testosterone. Younger men are not getting screened soon enough – as early as their thirties would be a good thing.

I have to remain positive for all those around me. I am positive for my children, I'm positive for my wife, and doing so makes me stronger and happier. I am not saying that I am always on the upper level of being positive. There are days when it all goes wrong and I struggle and it makes me think. A positive outlook is the key, I believe. Your mind controls your body. It's how you think, how you program yourself like a computer. My medical team told me that the day might come when my abiraterone medication will stop working, but there are other treatments out there, unlike years before. When that day comes, I will cross that bridge. I'm going to use the abiraterone until it stops working. I am not going to live like a hermit until then. I thank God each and every day that it has not been as bad as it could have been.

My inner voice stopped me from breaking down the day I was told I had cancer, five years ago. My inner voice to me is spiritual. A deeper understanding of the nature and function of my consciousness can help me feel in control of my own life and give meaning to my existence. I can control my consciousness even in my darkest moments.

The news was not good, but my head remained unbowed. I can only proclaim my strength in the face of adversity to that of 'I am the master of my fate: I am the captain of my soul,' words by the poet William Ernest Henley. I have been in control of my journey from the moment of diagnosis. Though at times I felt like that control was lost, it was only for a fleeting moment. I spend every moment of every day talking with my subconscious, asking it for advice, asking it all manner of questions. I suppose at times I hoped that it would be a two-way conversation, but alas this was not to be: the silent, inconclusive questions remained unanswered.

If I could roll the clock back to that point in time when my body became aware of cancer activating itself within, then my life would have been so different. With this said, we are now living in a time where the possibility of this happening is real. I am quite sure that my mother had the faulty gene and passed it on. It's been there all my life. Now that I have the ammunition of knowledge, I can inform my children. Knowing there is an abnormal gene in the family means that my children can be screened far earlier than they would be otherwise. That to me is a very good thing.

The future is exciting and full of real life-prolonging possibilities. How you feel changes how you act and as such influences your personality. I know that the thought process for me must vary from living with my condition to dealing with the possibility of dying.

When the body stops working properly, so does the brain in moments of poor health. Many people tend to think of the brain as somehow separate from the body, but it's really not so: even something as basic as diet can have a surprisingly large impact on our brain function and thus memory, thought processes and personality. Therefore, having the body shut down completely can really mess up the brain, causing hallucinations, disassociations, memory lapses, and reliving old memories.

It is estimated that at least 500,000 people living with and beyond cancer have one or more physical or psychosocial consequences of their cancer or its treatment, altering their lives on a long-term basis. My doctors say that remission is not possible, but that controlling and managing the cancer is. There is no cure for stage four prostate cancer at this moment in time. I fully understand that, but it does not stop me from thinking there may be in two or three years from now.

Many people with cancer experience short-term physical side effects during treatment, and usually these will resolve naturally within a few months. However, some will experience long-term or late-onset 'consequences of treatment' – the wide range of physical and psychosocial changes that reduce the quality of life after cancer and its treatment, no matter how long ago that treatment might have been administered. It is accepted that both short- and long-term consequences of treatment may occur as a result of the inevitable damage to normal tissues in the body when undertaking treatments that are designed to be highly destructive to cancer cells. It is also well known that there can be serious, long-lasting psychosocial effects.

However, it is less well known that problems can persist, or appear as new problems, years or even decades after treatment. I believe that people need a level of information about the risks of treatment and how to cope with problems when they arise. Certain cancer treatments increase the risk of long-term conditions such as heart disease, osteoporosis or a second cancer, and they can add other acute and chronic conditions common in older age, resulting in serious health and social care problems or premature death.

As I continue to write across the scars of pain and you read my words, it is my hope that you are empowered to believe that you too can make it through a cancer journey and understand the road I have travelled. I am at peace with myself now that I have written my words. I am a strong man getting stronger day by day. I am a man crying on the inside but not on the outside. My book is an eternal gift to the world of cancer patients. I am the same person, just a little older, fatter and wiser to the world around me. There were and still are moments during my journey when I cursed to the point that you could see the blue coming out of my mouth. I hope that my book, which is my fingerprint, will make an indelible mark on many people's lives. I walk with my head held high and a sense of purpose as my life becomes inextricable from the life of my cancer.

7: My secret storm

There have been so many occasions during these past five years that I have looked out of the windows by my home or hospital bed and raised my head up to the skies and watched the stormy weather pelt down on this earth. In doing so, I have likened the stormy weather conditions to my situation and my thought process, wanting to converse with the Almighty. You see, I was schooled to believe in the notion that there is a heavenly body that answers all prayers and questions.

Day after day I prayed to be healed; day after day I shed a tear as my illness tugged away at my physical structure and emotional heart strings, removing yet another day of my life on this place called Earth. Whilst my eyes gazed upon the storm created by nature, I did not take its presence to indicate the absence of the Almighty. Far from it; I realise that storms take different forms, ranging from health-related and physical to financial and emotional. In this instance, I am not talking about the storms that bring forth rain, hailstones, lightning or thunderstorms. I am talking about the personal life storms that other people cannot see. The undetectable storms that make people think that, in your everyday life, you are not subjected to hell. Just because I get out of my bed each and every morning, wash, dress and put on my mask then waltz into a room smiling, you think all is well.

Take a moment to think and reflect upon this; when confronted with a sand storm, what would be your first course of action? Would it not be to keep your head down and cover your face, eyes and keep your mouth shut? In doing so you then find you are unable to see anything around you because your head is down, praying for the sandstorm to pass. Similarly, when going through a visible storm, help, in more cases than not, is on hand; whether from a comfort, advisory or financial point of view, someone is aware of your situation. But when you are going through a secret storm it is exactly that, 'secret.' There's no comfort, there's no one there, just you and the secret storm that you are surrounded by. It becomes a very lonely place to dwell.

I do not believe for one moment that people in general have not gone through storms in their lives, because we all have them in one form or another. There are those who have gone through a secret storm and, in doing so, will understand what a cancer diagnosis means. In life, many people question atrocities of unbelievable proportions. I know I have. I have advanced metastatic prostate cancer and no amount of praying to the Almighty has changed my condition to that of a total cure. However, I still pray. I still believe that I will get through and to give up is not an option. It's moments like this that the biblical verse 2 Corinthians 5:7 KJV comes into its own – 'For we live by faith, not by sight.' My secret storm is ten-fold to what most of you have gone through and are no longer going through, unlike me, as I am still living this secret storm every day.

'I'm braver because I fought against a giant and won. I'm stronger because I had to be. I'm happier because I've learned what matters. I stand taller because I am a survivor.' But I still find that I revert back into my secret storm mode when my PSA test results loom. The simplest reason for this reversion is this: had I kept my eye on my health I would never have found myself in this position in the first place.

In life, sometimes we as men need a stark message/reminder to be set before us, sometimes the nagging wife, girlfriend or even a friend is not enough. Because, as is usual, we believe we are invincible, and nothing can touch us; well I am here to say that this is a myth. I was your typical 'alpha male', yet cancer touched me with a vengeance. Maybe if I had read the following words of the late Martin Luther King Jnr. I would have avoided much pain and anguish – 'Nothing in the world is more dangerous than sincere ignorance and conscientious stupidity.'

For most people with cancer today, treatment is administered in the outpatient setting – patients do not have to stay in hospital. This, in my opinion, is a wonderful situation to be in. I recall with eye-watering bitterness the time when my mother underwent her ordeal. I was scarred for life by what I saw and felt emotionally in that hospital,never stopping to think for one moment that one day I might have to endure the same.

Regardless of in-patient or out-patient situations, we often need some form of assistance and support to deal with an array of issues facing us, namely the side effects of the treatment we are undergoing and the psychological issues. The aim of all cancer treatment is to cure the person afflicted. Imagine an advanced cancer diagnosis such as mine, and living under the guise of being classed as 'cured' but never 'clear' as there is no guarantee that every cancer cell has been eliminated. All the medical team can say is that at the time of checking they found nothing in the blood test investigation. I liken it to flu and taking some sort of medication, which does not mean you will not get the same illness again at some stage down the line.

You can be classed as 'cured', as that is the aim of the treatment, but never deemed 'clear'. That is why we hear the term 'no evidence of disease' coined so often, even though it is not exactly the same situation.

For most of us, we just try to carry on with our lives as near to the new 'normal' that we have been introduced to and supposedly become accustomed to. Let me assure you, that this is easier said than done and this is why many sufferers end up going through a secret storm, not once, but many times.

I have seen better days, but I have also seen real bad days. I do not have everything I want in life, but I do have all I need. Waking up in the morning with aches and pains is the new norm for me, but at least I wake up. My life may not be perfect, but at least I now know that I am blessed with the strength to continue this battle. It is truly hoped that you too will find the strength to fight, to stand up tall and declare that you also are a victor, not a victim nor a prisoner.

8: *When a friend dies*

It was Thursday 24th September 2015 when I received a telephone call informing me that a friend had died. My friend, Gordon Holt, passed away in the early hours of Wednesday 23rd September. Gordon was diagnosed with leukaemia eleven years ago and, at that time, he was not given long to survive. But he did, and for eleven more years, he played a further part in many people's lives, including mine.

For me, when a friend dies, a part of you also dies. I knew my friend for thirty years and always enjoyed his banter, humour and company. For me, though, he played the greatest part in my life during the past four years. You see, I, like my friend, was also diagnosed with cancer in January 2012, primarily advanced metastatic prostate cancer. Like my friend, the unsavoury news was as shocking and 'Think short-term rather than long-term' were the words given to me by my doctor. Shocked, bewildered and lost, I turned to the only person I knew who could and would understand what I was about to go through – Gordon, my friend.

In the early years of my disease, when I was going up and down through life's hills and valleys and I thought that there was no way out, my friend was there for me. During our first few conversations, he listened with compassion, empathy, and care. Even moments of silence were not awkward, and that was the start of many, many conversations between us. I found in him the real meaning of a friend that so many so-called friends lacked and could never aspire to be. He had an ear to bend and he would listen to my trials, tribulations and woes.

We, the people with life-limiting diseases, find ourselves agonisingly lonely in dealing with our illness and the fight for life as we pace up and down on a daily basis in our homes. Cancer, that dreaded C word, is the most feared word in any language, the disease that affects many different parts of the body and in ways some of which are more serious than others. The many faces of this disease challenge an individual to show their fighting spirit and their will and determination to live. My friend certainly showed all of these traits.

When I was talking with my friend, he showed me a heroic attitude and mindset that bordered on that of any kind of elite Special Forces soldier, oblivious to the dangers of his condition and a fighter amongst fighters. His weapons were faith, determination, and loads of guts.

I recall our talks with eye-watering bitterness. 'Alf,' he once said, 'I have decided that I am going to enjoy what life I have left and travel with my wife to different places around the world that I have not been to. Not sure how I'm going to fund it but that's what I'm going to do.' My friend fulfilled all that he said to me and more; he became my hero. He would call me upon his return from various places and tell me snippets about these visits and then change the subject mid-flow and ask, 'So what about you – how you doing, Alf?' You see, after sitting alone on a daily basis with no one to talk to about my condition, or more importantly, about how I was feeling, it was as if God himself had spoken to me.

Not until you have walked in my shoes and felt my pain will you understand what any cancer patient or survivor ever undergoes, but my friend did. If you don't believe me, visit the special group chat rooms on Facebook where you will see the special bonds being created that are helping people with life-threatening and life-limiting diseases. The void Gordon left will never ever be filled.

Gordon was a white Jewish guy whose claim to fame was that he had worked in Electric Avenue in Brixton, south London, the heart of the Caribbean community in the 1960s and scene of the notorious riots in the 1970s. He sported a large afro hairstyle, which he was so proud of, and replayed the same stories amongst others, oh so many times, but they never got old. I found that we connected culturally, and his sense of humour always prevailed regardless of his circumstances.

When you are down on your knees, sometimes it is fun moments like these that allow you as an individual not only to see the funny side of matters but also to forget about your ailments for a moment. Even if it's just for a moment, that's all we who are sick need to touch base with normality. The blood tests, the medication, the fatigue and the sickness are just some of the lifestyles imposed upon us by this unwanted illness. Friendships come, friendships go, but ours was special; colour and creed were not barriers and we openly talked about the woes and ills of the world, as I too had travelled the world in my professional capacity.

The sadness I feel within me at his loss clouded my eyes today at his funeral as I reminisced on previous conversations, especially when his son read a wonderful eulogy that his father would have been proud of; I know I was. I also know that, as time moves along, reminders and triggers of our friendship will flash through my mind and open floodgates of emotion and memories, but I know that these were of the kind that aided me in my illness and, as such, were better than any medication that a human being could take to feel better. Maybe we should have bottled what we had going and given it away for free to all those who did not have what we had. Those reading this right now will, at the very least, gain an insight into why friendships are extremely important during illness.

I will not need any special way to remember my friend, such as birthdays, anniversaries or otherwise. Our friendship is firmly etched in my mind. I grieved today when you were laid to rest, Gordon; my eyes, hidden by dark glasses, were red, puffed and watery, but from here on in my thoughts will always be that we celebrated the highs and were there to support each other during the lows. I have shared a bit of me with all of you reading my blog; however, remember we all need meaningful connections with other people – after all, we never need to be or feel alone in this world.

'Share honest appreciation of a friend every chance you get.'

9: Overcoming adversity

I have always felt that in the face of this terrible adversity I have been positive throughout. But what was it that aided me and made me believe in myself so that I could get through? They say God helps those that help themselves; this is something that sounds like truth. Many days and nights I sat pondering and asking myself what stuff I am made of. What am I really made of? Then the push came and I found what lay at the very core of my character. This was when I learnt what I was made of and who I was as a person.

One of the biggest challenges we humans face is adversity. Whether we like it or not, adversity is a part of everyday life. Overcoming it is one of the biggest hurdles we face. The English writer and physician Havelock Ellis wrote that 'Pain and death are part of life. To reject them is to reject life itself.' Problems, whether big or small, present themselves throughout our entire existence. Regardless of your status in life, you will encounter struggles, challenges, hardship and, at times, heart-wrenching moments.

At this moment in time, I am facing the greatest adversity of my life: cancer. But does this make my adversity different from Peter, David or Joan's? Hell no. Throughout my life, I have faced all sorts of adversities and learned how to deal with and overcome them all. I firmly believe that doing so steadied me for what I am now undergoing. It is this that built my character and resilience. All the challenges and difficulties I confronted and overcame in life served to strengthen my will, determination, confidence and ability to conquer obstacles ahead, such as prostate cancer.

Herodotus, the Greek historian, said, 'Adversity has the effect of drawing out strength and qualities of a man that would have lain dormant in its absence.' For me, this awakening roused and stirred emotions of war-like nature as I prepared myself like a soldier prepares for war. As I responded positively and constructively to the character and perseverance merged deep inside of me, I was truly on course for the war of wars – me versus cancer. If only it could have realised that my inner strength matched it in ferocity and strength, it may have gone somewhere else instead. As with anything, once the mindset was going through a learning curve, at first I found myself entangled in self-pity, the unfairness of life. I ask, Why me? And in doing so I did not recognise that there existed the opportunities for wisdom and growth that walk hand in hand with adversity.

As is the case with most things in life, 'Time is the master' – which was something that I had plenty of opportunities to experience. As the misty haze lifted from my vision, I started to think far more clearly. In doing so, I set adrift the self-defeating and unproductive thoughts and got down to living and dealing with the matter before me.

I had learned the valuable lesson that to avoid or resist adversity was only to allow it to persist. Wherever you look in the world today, there is an unmistakable struggle, with tsunami floods and calamities of all types befalling mankind. Even within my own circle of family and friends, there was death, loss, and tragedy. Pain is inevitable in this world; however, suffering is optional.

Overcoming adversity should be one of our main challenges in life. When we resolve to confront and overcome it, we become expert at dealing with it and consequently triumph over our day-to-day struggles. When things go wrong and we tumble, life shows us that it is a continuous succession of highs and lows, of small and large problems that never end. As soon as you overcome one problem you are besieged by another. Sometimes you are hit by simultaneous problems at once. It's called life – two steps forward, one step back.

And if you think it gets any easier, then think again. The bigger and wealthier you become, the more you just exchange one type of problem for another – and these have enormous consequences as opposed to your previous limited consequences.

You will have noticed that I rarely use the word 'cancer', as a means of escapism for my dilemma. It should be self-evident from what I have written that those of you suffering from cancer have already unknowingly prepared for our greatest adversity. No matter how smart and clever you are, you will face struggles, challenges, difficulties and sometimes heart-breaking adversities every day, week and month of your life. As a result, you are the person you are today. When you contend with hard times beyond your strength to handle, you become this person and will continue to be this new person who is positive in the face of this terrible adversity.

I am saddened when I see or hear about people giving up without realising that they have in fact already passed through this realm of adversity. A critical ailment such as advanced metastatic prostate cancer should not send one into panic mode. The starting point in dealing with any difficulty is to simply relax, focus, clear your mind and try and be in full control of your emotions and senses. Without this process you have failed before you start. You have to develop an alternative to that which you face, or you will become anxious and maybe panicky as you are threatened with this reversal to an area of your life. Think of it this way: people who are successful in life are not without life's problems. They, however, are people who respond quickly and positively to their problems.

When talking with my family I had to define the worst possible outcome that could happen as a result of my diagnosis of stage four prostate cancer and possible death. Kissing the hand of the Almighty was not the answer – it was concentrating on channelling all my energies towards ensuring the very worst did not happen. One should remember that many issues regarding adversities arise because of misunderstandings and incorrect information sought or supplied from a third party. Ask yourself, who do I know that may have had this disease? Also, ask how they managed to deal with it and survive. You should never be afraid to ask around; we were all blind at the initial stage of diagnosis. A positive affirmation that springs to mind comes from the motivational speaker Les Brown, as he looks at the problems of life that we face and he states, 'It has not come to stay; it has come to pass.' Whatever it is, and however difficult it may appear, say to yourself, 'It will pass.' No matter what happens, never ever give up.

10: *A viewpoint on cancer and beliefs*

Around the world, substantial numbers of people are diagnosed with cancer each and every day: some will die, while others will survive. Upon diagnosis, each of these people is plunged into a dark tunnel that will change their lives dramatically, some for the short term, others over a longer period. Faced with an apparently endless chain of medical tests, examinations, second opinions, medications, surgery, new tests, supportive therapies, and follow-up checks, they find themselves at the complete mercy of the disease. Crawling through that dark tunnel, each patient feeds into an immense medical apparatus that employs millions of people and generates billions and billions of dollars in revenue for the medical and pharmaceutical industries.

To the medical profession, I say this: you do indeed perform some amazing life-saving procedures, but you still have your head buried in the sand when it comes to cancer. To the pharmaceutical industry, I also say that you have indeed saved countless lives, but you remain wilfully ignorant of proven alternative treatments. You cannot argue or otherwise disprove.

A few years ago, I received the news that I had stage four prostate cancer. My doctor told me to think short term rather than long term. My interpretation of this statement was that I had months to live.

As I fought this horrendous disease, I realised that I needed some heavenly help. As I usually do when I'm in trouble, I talked to the Spiritual Being above, and in doing so, I made a deal.

I told the Spiritual Being that if He would help me through this, I would become a beacon of light for those who are ignorant to (in my case) prostate cancer as well as those who are suffering and riddled with the disease. Well, a deal is a deal. It was not an instant change on my part, as nothing necessarily happens in a day. A few weeks later, I visited with Pastor Stephen Ramos, who told me that he had spoken with God a few months before I was hospitalised and that God had told him that I would be healed and that I would come out stronger and fitter. However, Pastor Ramos then continued, telling me he had asked God again the question 'Will this man be healed?' The answer came back that 'I have told you already that this man will be OK.' This was the last discussion that I ever had with Pastor Ramos, an angel who had been sent to deliver me a message. Pastor Ramos died two weeks later of a brain aneurysm. What made this so important was that he had travelled half way across London to deliver this message to me personally in my hospital bed.

I agree that medication played a part in my healing process, but my religious belief played a far greater and stronger role. I was healed because of Pastor Ramos's message from God.

We all believe in and accept something as we travel through life, no matter how small or big that belief is. We hang on to a belief without empirical evidence, and in doing so we are guided to an eventual destination. For some of us, that destination is good; for others, not so good. Grit, determination, hope, love, and emotions are not medicines but rather attributes within a person. These attributes, in the grand scheme of things, greatly overshadow the powers of the medical and pharmaceutical industries.

One would not be wrong to categorise this as a fatalistic belief, depending on your point of view. There is nothing fatalistic in believing the word of the ultimate Spiritual Being we call God.

There are many people out there, people who believe that 'almost everything causes cancer.' Fewer believe that 'there's not much people can do to lower their chances of getting cancer.' Other points of view are that 'there is so much advice about preventing cancer that it's hard to know which ones to follow.'

However, the reality is that cancer, for most, comes with a high monetary cost, and there is another way to combat cancer that doesn't come with a price tag: faith in God, ultimately not tied to any particular religion. For me, people who believe in a higher being tend to show better physical function and more responsiveness to cancer treatment.

Everyone's cancer journey differs, but ultimately we listen for the recognisable cancer survival words – think remission. You see, cancer is tricky like that: just when you think the horizon is clear, it can creep up on you again like a thief in the night. But we still have one thing – our belief – and cancer can't take that away from us no matter what else it strips us of. No matter what, our belief remains intact.

For me, culture is a fundamental part of one's being. Spirituality is integrated with culture and both play a significant role in a person's journey through life. Yet culture and spirituality are often misunderstood and may not seem to be important in healthcare settings. I suggest that for us adults with cancer and families, this should not be ignored.

11: Making adjustments

I know that cancer is an illness that changes so much, and takes control of life in ways that most people could never imagine. However, having gone through it, I believe the one thing you do get to choose is how you approach the illness. We have an incredible amount of choice in what we do and how we behave. The old adage that 'attitude is everything' applies very well to the battle that one is required to wage against cancer. But while you are going through it, it's hard just to face the day that lies before you, let alone face the days that are to follow. It's even harder to face the fact that you may not be here for the dates and plans that you hear other people discussing.

This life-limiting disease that you are going through requires you to make serious adjustments in your life and lifestyle. If your lifestyle was somewhat manic and hectic, you will find the changes hard to accept, and even harder to implement. Stress is a major factor in life in general, and, as such, must be managed well in all disciplines. It goes without saying that reducing your stress levels, living a balanced life, and taking good care of yourself will ensure your existence on this earth for a little while longer. It is clear as to what stress does to a human being, besides raising one's blood pressure to the point of bringing on a possible stroke. One life-threatening illness is bad enough; tempting fate with another is ill-advised. 'Just let whatever is stressing you go' is easier said than done at times, but your life depends on it. Look at it this way: a moment of madness could be a lifetime of misery. Let it pass, let it go; it's just not worth your time or effort.

Try not to take your work home, and make time for loved ones more frequently. Money is not the be-all and end-all in life. Take time out to smell the roses and enjoy your life. So many of us were, and are, so busy making a living that we forget how to live. Has that not been the story of many who have fallen before us? For those who have kept relatively fit, you will understand the frame of mind that it places you in and the effect on your body and mind.

Taking care of you must be a priority. I recall the neuropathy pains that were tingling through my feet; regular walking and some stretching stopped these pains in their tracks. The minute I stopped stretching, however, they came back. Not for an instance am I saying we are all in the same boat where prostate cancer is concerned, but allowing your body to stiffen up and neuropathy pains to prevail will definitely play havoc with your mind.

One of the things in life that I enjoy is eating out. However, I used to overindulge in foods such as burgers, red meat, ice cream and other fatty foods, which are now a thing of the past for me. I now have to control my eating habits far better these days. Thankfully, most restaurants these days have their menus online, so I am able to see what foods suit my lifestyle before I leave my home. 'You are what you eat.' Clearly having menus online minimises the stress of going somewhere and not being able to choose something from the menu that suits your new lifestyle.

By thinking smart and eating smart, you can still enjoy your life regardless of what you are facing. By monitoring your actions you can track your behaviours and progress, which helps you and your oncology team far better. Yes, it can be outright boring to keep notes and graphs, but from a mental perspective, just imagine seeing your graphical plot moving towards a healthier outlook through your own endeavours and discipline.

Finally, I have learnt like many others that not everyone around you is conducive to your betterment, and that also includes family members. Establish a support network system around you that will allow you to maintain healthy relationships. These should be people who totally understand what you are going through and have your best interests at heart at all times. Keep away from people who are blood-sucking vampires or leeches. In reality, you will find that they are few and far between.

I was extremely fortunate to have a wonderful friend and wife before I took ill, and she has supported me throughout every aspect of my illness. When I was financially impaired she propped me up until I could stand on my two feet again. When I was in pain she soothed and comforted me until it was a distant memory. When those who did not mean me well came around me she acted as my personal bodyguard and bared her teeth like a tigress protecting her young. God help anyone who dared to enter her lair, with her sharpened teeth ready to bite. She spared no one including so-called family and friends. Although she was one in a million, I have to say there were many horror stories that I have heard first-hand from other sufferers about partners or wives walking out on them or making unreasonable demands on them. What is it about people who profess their love for another human being under the eyes of God and the Church only to show their inhumanity towards them? I just cannot get my head around that at all. I really can't.

I have referred to my mother's passing on many occasions throughout my book. The death of a loved one is not only a loss; it is a turning point. The world will never be the same again. Having been through this traumatic experience I am well placed to understand how a bereaved person feels as they face long periods of adjustment to a life which is seldom wanted or planned. As a result, there were social implications placed before me and, as such, adjustments in life had to be made. But quickly the recognition of my mother's cancer journey was just becoming that of mine as the physical, psychological, emotional, behavioural and spiritual symptoms all started to have an impact.

It is an absolute minefield when you start to weigh all that is against you, and the adjustments required are rather daunting.

The **physical symptoms** include pain, nausea, sleep disturbance, mobility, fatigue, lack of coordination, and constipation.

Psychological/emotional: moodiness, irritability, depression, guilt complex, sadness, bouts of crying, frustration, anxiety, fear and anger.

Behavioural symptoms: poor concentration, forgetfulness, slower thinking and loss of confidence.

Spirituality: Intense spiritual search, rejection of previous beliefs and practices, anger at God, fear of judgment and questions about the meaning of life.

Losses: employment, financial status, sexual life/intimacy, and future dreams (seeing my children and grandchildren grow up).

Social Implications: fear of being alone, drifting away to you own thoughts during conversations, and abruptness with people.

As I stated earlier, serious adjustments are required in your life to enable you to change and move on. If I am, to be honest, I have not even achieved half of these because the reality is that it's near impossible. So my wife and I just try to do the best that we can under the circumstances and if a reversal of an adult to a child happens (start learning all over again), then the theory of retrogenesis – 'once a man, twice a child' – becomes factual.

Alfred Samuels

12: Don't put off because of cancer

As a cancer sufferer, I have often thought about the times I have
walked my own green mile. But as time progressed, I decided that I
was not going to wait anymore until I was looking good on paper because
I may not ever be 100% cancer-free on paper. Whilst frustrating, these
thoughts and constant daily changes in my health have taught me the
importance of living my life.

I enjoy doing things when I can. I no longer wait. I try not to put things
off anymore, because I know I may never feel 100%. If I feel good enough,
I go ahead and do something.

The one thing, though, that I would advise any new cancer patient is
to get an advocate, a person who will ask questions and do the necessary
research. When I was tired or just not in the right headspace, having an
advocate allowed me to just be an ordinary patient. 'Sometimes you just
aren't going to feel like it' – it was at times like that that I counted on my
own advocate. My wife.

When I was first diagnosed more than four years ago, the statistics
weren't encouraging. If I had allowed the data and figures to influence
my mind when I was first diagnosed, I wouldn't be here. So rather than

worrying about these statistics, I just stayed focused on the future. There were the usual specific things I kept my sight on, such as family and business, but helping others and forgetting about my own ailment became first and foremost. That's what I saw on the horizon. With the support of my family, I have tried not to allow cancer to deny me those things.

I am not as fortunate as some who have gone through active cancer treatment – for now, that is. As I look enviously at my family enjoying summer holidays and excursions, I have to admit, yet again, that I am somewhat jealous. I have my moments when I try not to focus on holidays or short travel breaks, but instead see new places, have new experiences and make memories rather than acquiring and maintaining 'stuff'.

I understand the need to prioritise my medical appointments during holidays. However, the more I age, the quicker time seems to be slipping by. I want to live my priorities rather than getting pulled down by my 'stuff'. I find that I am getting more bogged down with other things these days. Instead of planning and taking much-needed recuperation, I am putting it back. October 2014 was our last holiday, and since then both our minds and bodies have gone through a lot and now require the much-needed vitamin D. Back, back, back, until 'later' or 'next year' doesn't happen. Now I am consciously aware of this danger.

I have learned that holidays float within a very short window of opportunity. I don't just want to travel with my wife on holidays but also with my kids. They are no longer babies; they are totally self-sufficient and, as such, attention to their whims is no longer required.

For me, the older they get, the more they enjoy the same stuff that Mum and Dad enjoy. Oh, how I just want to enjoy sitting on the beach with my wife, daughters and sons and talk about the past and maybe even the future. I also want to travel more with them before they are far too busy with jobs and activities, while they are able to enjoy my company and while I am still around.

I have travelled extensively throughout the world as an adult, primarily for work-related reasons, without much time for husband-and-wife vacations, let alone a family vacation. If I am honest, I can count on both of my hands the time devoted to holidays past, and I do not feel happy about this but needs must. My wife and I work. We work. And we work. I feel, and I know, that my wife feels the need to untie the knots in our bodies and clear the haze from our minds that we have spent months creating. Simplify! Take that holiday now!

As a survivor, I ask myself what I would regret if I or someone in my family were to die suddenly. Especially as an advanced cancer survivor, one of my regrets would be not having travelled and vacationed more with those dear to me. There are always trade-offs. Would I wish I had foregone a three- to six-month work contract for an adventure? Since I can't take my stuff with me when my time is up, the priority boils down to relationships and life experiences, which include seeing the sights this world has, and sharing those experiences with friends and family while I am here to do so.

I know I am great at getting stuck in a rut and bogged down in routine.

Travel is sometimes a much-needed break from the routine. Visiting new places and trying new activities is an opportunity to learn and think 'outside the box.' It is sad that sometimes people move, change marital partners or switch jobs when all they really may have needed was a holiday, a break and a refreshed perspective on life. I have often wondered why my wife put up with my work lifestyle. I know my children hated it, and as they got older they voiced their opinions.

I like the anticipation of travel plans. Although my wife is the one to organise everything, I throw in my penny's worth just to feel unalienated from the process. Well, that's what I tell myself. A Caribbean cruise or European romantic hotspots are places that we are enthusiastic about. Exceedingly long-haul trips are not something we favour because it causes me so much discomfort if I am not in Business or First class. Financially, that's something out of our range. Clearly, if we won the lottery then to experience that would be wonderful, having personally experienced it from a work perspective. The one thing we always did while on holiday was to laugh more. Something I can only say I wish I could do more of regardless of my situation.

Every trip has an end; it's good to come back home. As the saying goes, 'There's no place like home.' It's sad that our little trip is over, but all good things come to an end. I no longer take our budding trees, lakes and nearby picturesque canal for granted. Travel shows us options, yet it also deepens our appreciation for what we already have – things we are quick to take for granted when engaged in the daily grind of life.

Consider what your priorities are and what the windows of opportunity for them are. My window of opportunity is today. Am I going to think about it and talk about it, or am I going to do it? When are you going to take that vacation? Some memories are better made sooner rather than later. What trips and adventures are on your bucket list?

I want to live by my motto of 'Don't wait to live' – just make the most of your life now.

13: The importance of a super-positive attitude

According to medical statistics, one in three westerners will be diagnosed with cancer at some point. Within five years of their diagnosis, at least one of these three people will die from their cancer. Fortunately, medical advances in cancer treatments have allowed nearly fifty per cent of patients to eventually be cured. In other words, these patients will live more than five years after first being diagnosed.

Patients who have their cancer detected early and go through successful cancer surgery have the highest chance of living more than five years after their diagnosis. The reason I know this is true is that I am a cancer patient myself and I've already surpassed the milestone of five years.

After I was diagnosed, I questioned whether I would even survive for five years. Of course, it helped that I possessed the traits of someone who could survive this first cancer milestone. Not only was I getting the best treatment imaginable, but I was young and had a lot to live for in this world. When it came to figuring out the information about my treatment, I understood all of it and was motivated to follow through.

I've gone through all the turmoil and harsh feelings that people with cancer commonly experience, such as anger, fear, uncertainty, shock, despair and vulnerability. These are feelings that will cause you to lose your appetite and give you symptoms of depression and insomnia. And when you consider the side effects of the medication I was given, this just added feelings of disorientation and fatigue into the mix.

In my heart, I know that my positivity was what saved my life. Over the last five years, having a positive attitude has gotten me and my family through the difficult times of dealing with the advanced metastatic prostate cancer that I've suffered from. If it weren't for this positivity, I'm sure I wouldn't be alive today. I was even able to stay positive after learning that medical statistics revealed that having a positive attitude cannot make cancer patients live longer. Obviously, I strongly disagree with this. Anyone who researches modern medical literature regarding their cancer will see there is a reason to have hope. That's how it was for me. After researching advanced metastatic prostate cancer, the one thing that was abundantly clear was that it was incurable. After the initial shock wore off, I stayed sitting at my computer for a good thirty minutes with a big smile on my face. All I could think was, now the battle begins. It was as if I had the mindset of an army general who was about to lead his troops into battle.

Next, I underwent a protocol for experimental treatment that consisted of a special drug trial programme. Over the last five years, I had to go to a cancer treatment centre every eight weeks for a meeting with my oncology team so they could give me a prostate medical review. This included both the PSA and my blood results. These demanding clinical trial programmes made the patients act like partners of the clinic. After all, these clinical trials involve a lot of time, testing and travel by the patient, which can be quite frustrating. However, I do think that clinical trials need to be friendlier to the patients because they can leave a patient feeling like they're trapped in a rigid orderly environment.

As I approached my fifth year of treatment for prostate cancer, the readings of my regular PSA recordings were less than 0.1 nanograms per millilitre. All my other blood levels were equally normal. With any luck, I shall reach the second milestone of ten years after first being diagnosed with cancer. The gift that I have received is the gift of time, which is totally priceless. This gave me the ability to think, plan, and fight.

Statistics have never gone over well in my mind. The only purpose they serve is for fulfilling my goal, which is remission. If I'm going to keep moving forward and extend my time on this earth, I need only positive statements in my life. After shedding tears, sweat, and blood trying to get to this state of mind, I am happy to say that I've finally gotten there.

I am still optimistic about going forward as I draw inspiration from my inner emotions and my willingness to help other people in my situation. Scientists just don't understand the concept of thinking long term rather than short term. Of course, every person is physically and emotionally devastated when they're first diagnosed with cancer. But it is how we move forward that determines whether cancer wins or we win.

Of course, I am not deluding myself into thinking that I don't have cancer anymore, because I do. I have not gone into full remission yet and until I do, cancer will still be holding me hostage. When I look back on my life, I realise that I didn't pay enough attention to my health because I was so busy working and trying to make a living I forgot how to live. I wish I had done more actual 'living' during those years.

I am a firm believer that attitude has a lot to do with survival, even though the medical community does not believe this. If you've never had cancer before, try to think outside of the box for a minute. Imagine having a serious medical condition like prostate cancer and having to spend every waking moment literally fighting for your life. You have to be dependent on regular intravenous and oral medication, even though there is some toxicity in the medication and it destroys the functionality of your organ tissue. However, you still remain positive and optimistic regardless of these circumstances. The strength you have internally and mentally is what allows you to be this way.

It is possible to make positive changes in your life after getting diagnosed with cancer. It is possible to overcome adversity. It is possible to have hope. Again, cancer survivors are still going to have all kinds of emotional reactions inside of them caused by their disease. But it's our strong internal senses that allow us to move forward.

Also, it is normal for us and our families to start feeling demoralised, depressed, and isolated over the situation. Between the threat of mortality and the drastic changes that take place in our lives, it can be very stressful and distressing. Anytime someone goes through feelings like this, it can cause us to reflect on the meaning of life and the purpose we serve in this world. Self-reflecting over our own lives and goals will also take place, which can be painful at first but then lead to positive changes in your life.

We all want to disprove the statistics by using our willpower and determination to rebel against them. I would not be alive right now if I hadn't constructed positive mental thoughts to keep myself afloat. If you give up these positive thoughts for a statistic that is separate from your own mind and inner emotions, cancer will win for sure. It is easy to want to give up when faced with a difficult situation, which is all the more reason why positivity needs to be consistent in your mind.

The fact that I am alive today just proves statistics are misguided, negative and usually inaccurate. Statistics had shown that I was probably going to die within five years, but then I ended up living past that. This is proof that statistics cannot be trusted and why anyone fighting cancer should keep themselves as far away from statistical information as possible.

There aren't too many people who understand statistics to know what they truly mean. Instead, we just look at the statistics and immediately take them to heart. When I was told that I only had six months left to live, based on statistics, I did not want to believe it – and I never did believe it. Five years later, I can honestly say that positivity led me to this point.

It took me a long time to realise that I wasn't the only person affected by my diagnosis. My friends, family, and wife also became victims.

I started a regime of personal healing inspired by the philosophies of traditional herbal medicines from the Caribbean and the newest medical research of the West. One time, a friend of a friend had been diagnosed with prostate cancer and he decided to use only traditional herbal medicines and no modern-day medicines. Unfortunately, this decision ended up costing him his life because the herbal medicines failed. When I heard this story, I knew I didn't want to make the same mistake that he did. I truly am thankful to my friend for sharing that story and getting me out of my state of immense confusion.

During my treatment journey I made important lifestyle changes, such as gradually disengaging myself from my international security career, at which I worked full-time. All I want to do now is share my experiences of cancer with other people who are in the same boat. Most importantly, I don't want people to cower in the corner when they see statistics that tell them they're going to die soon. If people can learn to stand up against these statistics and stay motivated to recover, then anything is possible.

I am thankful to still be alive and moving my body forward every single day. I know there are other people throughout the world who are struggling with cancer just like I was. I also know that beating cancer doesn't take a plethora of resources or high priced doctors. It takes positive beliefs and the willingness to want to live. I have always been an optimistic person who sees the glass half full rather than half empty.

If I am unable to go into remission, then I will be happy to live past eighty years of age and am thankful for each day I live during this time. If cancer diagnostics and treatment are new to you, then educate yourself so you can live and fight cancer every single day. Perhaps you won't survive long enough for a cure to be available, but you can still live a long life to eighty or even ninety years old. Doesn't that sound worth fighting for?

14: You don't know

Sometimes I feel that I'm wasting my time in life looking for others to understand my side, my story, my journey. I know I almost touched the other side during my illness, as I experienced venturing down the supposed end-of-life tunnel, feeling that those passed were waiting for me at the other end. But that night it was not to be, as my spirit was not yet ready to be released from my human body. I often pray to be released from this long-term illness so that I no longer feel the pain, suffering or anguish that this disease has caused my body.

However, right now I just feel I'm standing still in life's vicious circle as I try to make everyone understand what I am going through. I have learned forgiveness and acceptance, but sometimes it's hard to really apply these feelings to those near and dear. My family and friends are on the outside, whilst I'm on the inside. Things, I'm sure, look so much better from the outside, having once been there. It's 3am, you don't know all the things I go through: bursting out in a profuse sweat on my head and face. You don't know... feeling low; you don't know... feeling bad; you don't know... feeling emotional. You don't know and you say you understand the other side. You, my friends and family, all think you know and understand my current life.

Next time you look in the mirror, observe how when you approach it, your image becomes clearer. Now you are beginning to see the other side, and you can't touch it – but I did. I am so tired. Sometimes I feel like I just want to go home; sometimes I feel like I just need to go home. I'm closing my eyes again. Now it's 4am and that 'you don't know' moment (which will be back) just passed so maybe I can get some sleep. As I lay in my bed next to my partner I often wonder if she has one eye open monitoring my every movement and moment. Only she can really, truly understand the 'you don't know' moments. I wish everybody else did.

Often I wonder what their excuse will be tomorrow; I know what their excuse was today and it will probably be the same the day after for not helping someone with cancer in some small way. Too many excuses, too many things to do in your day, not even 15 minutes to spare a loved one. So little time left to make amends as darkness descends and the trumpet sounds as they lower away another dear one lost to the dust of the earth. Now that I am departed I am no longer a glancing thought in your mind and busy days, but I'll be thinking about you wherever I may be, and it will be your turn one day to go through 'you don't know' moments.

What is it about mankind that makes people so cruel to one another? The proverbial statement 'man to man is so unjust' springs to mind. I am intrigued by the lack of humanity and fellowship to another especially as I was brought up to believe that 'all men are created equally'. Careful research of this sweeping statement, though, suggests otherwise; it was never said, it was distorted and there for me lieth the issue – a misinterpretation of a biblical proverb. I am sure there will be those who would wish to correct me and show otherwise but the fact remains biblical passages use different languages in their interpretation but nowhere does it actually say 'man to man is so unjust'.

A sermon, a burial, a gathering and then you sit amongst others telling them what a wonderful man or father he was, but deep down inside full of remorse and guilt. I only wanted 15 minutes of your time when I was alive. You don't have to be a scientist or an academic researcher of human nature to know that is a true statement, you just have to live amongst humans and experience life for a period of time to understand. Well, you understand that humans are complex, just not necessarily understand human behaviour! The complexity of human behaviour is such that at times it feels like relying on the dipstick to understand the complexity of the internal combustion engine as one gets their hands dirty amid the mess. Do I have time for of all this? 'Hell no', this one is best suited to that human behavioural specialist. I'll just sit back and read the academic reports published but still, I know I won't ever understand. Takes me back to my school days trying to understand homo sapiens and sapiens and the ideological suggestion that skull head sizes dictated the brainier of the two. I mean, who dreams these things up!

Anyway, we have veered off course somewhat so let's get back on track. Time and energy expended on this are not what someone with cancer will or should do; I suppose I was having a bit of a rant and blowing off steam. You see mentally in my head space I remember being subjected to this kind of behaviour; you think I would have passed it, but in reality, I have not because that's just human behaviour and still you don't know.

15: A viewpoint on 'chemo brain'

Defined by the Oxford Dictionary as 'an organ of soft nervous tissue contained in the skull of vertebrates, functioning as the coordinating centre of sensation and intellectual and nervous activity', the brain is very complex. The term 'chemo brain' (sometimes also known as 'chemo fog') is a common term used by us cancer survivors to describe lapses in thinking and issues with memory, both of which can occur during and after cancer treatment. When I was first affected, I thought I was going mad: I also had numbness in my feet and hands, though not to the point of dropping things.

As a business owner, I found all this had a huge impact on my life, as I ran into problems processing information, thinking, remembering things, and paying attention. I was at the top of my profession in the security industry, but soon I found myself turning down work because of this chemo brain. The pill form of chemo (abiraterone) then caused disaster to strike financially, and my business slowly died in front of my eyes.

I had good days, when I was as sharp as a needle, and then there were days when I stared blankly at the computer and forgot how to do basic tasks. Forgetting the names of things was a regular occurrence, but I never forgot faces. I suppose different parts of my brain were affected, such as the memory retention cord versus the visual retention cord. I was totally frustrated when I was not able to get my words out to describe things. At times I would stare out into space hoping and wanting that missing word to drift by. It was always silly stuff like 'fork' or the name of a soft drink that I was used to drinking. Then there was the embarrassment in front of friends as I struggled to find simple, easy words to describe parts of a conversation that we were having. I was always totally aware of the piercing eyes that were watching my every action and listening to my every word.

During 2015 I had my first motivational speaking engagement, during which I tried to memorise four simple words as part of my speech. I found that I beat myself up mentally over this issue, but then I managed to get through by just simply talking from my heart, winning me a standing ovation. Crazy, isn't it? Simple worked in this case. In retraining the mind to combat and deal with this situation I found writing was one solution, along with Bikram yoga and saunas, these being places of solitude where one sits and meditates on practices of peacefulness and body relaxation, allowing for a possible better memory retention.

Physical exercise was another favourite of mine. I would walk up hills with a weighted backpack, though at times fatigue did become an issue. They say puzzles and learning a new language can be advantageous, but for me, I could never see the reasons why. Puzzles just added to the confused state I was already in, and as for learning new languages, I was having enough problems understanding English again, let alone trying to pronounce and utter a different language. Languages were just never my thing anyway.

Trying to multi-task was a definite no: just focusing on one thing at a time made more sense, and it worked but slowed down my day. As time moved on, I tried not to focus on how much these symptoms were bothering me: I just accepted it so that I was able to deal with it. For some of us, just laughing at it was a way out. I mean, haven't we all forgotten to do something in our lives? Taking the grocery list with us to the supermarket or some other strange thing from a mental perspective that made us laugh afterwards. Well, haven't we?

Keeping a diary I found very useful, because it allowed me to write however I wanted, often in shorthand that only I understood, and this worked well for me.

Clearly, the medical profession does not have the answers for the side effects of this chemo treatment we undergo. More research is needed in order to assist patients during and after the treatments. This debilitating condition is not a joke: it's our life that has been turned upside down, and that's nothing to laugh about.

Many friends and family don't even believe me when I talk about this condition. For those that understand, I think that when they suggest things to help, they aren't trying to minimise things. Still, there isn't a treatment yet for this aspect, and losing your business, your job, or social interaction is always devastating.

I can't get the right words out: I can't spell well, type well, or do mathematics the way I used to do. I have pain from head to toe, brutal neuropathy along with the rest. Crying outbursts at inappropriate times for no reason. I wish I knew how to recover from all of this and regain my quality of life. I can't wave a magic wand and rid myself of cancer. I am lucky to be alive and for that I am extremely grateful!

16: *Playing the hand the best way you know*

Cancer today is the biggest disease on the cultural map, bigger than Aids, cystic fibrosis or spinal injury, bigger even than those more prolific killers of men – heart disease and strokes. Prostate cancer is the second most commonly diagnosed cancer among men.

Nobody knows what a man goes through when he's diagnosed with prostate cancer, except the man himself. It's like being hit head on by a bus: getting up and walking away as if it hadn't happened simply isn't possible.

As the initial shock and fear set in, many people try to beat the illness with a positive attitude. Of course, you must take some time to let what has happened sink in. As you soak it all in, however, do not stand there too long. Be diligent as you move past the shock of the diagnosis. Your road may be a long one, it may be a short one, and it may be a network of spaghetti-like motorways that requires the patience of a Buddhist monk. You will forge your own path.

The mind and body will undergo much suffering, including side effects of the medications and treatments you undergo. You will go through an undetermined period of major emotional and physical strain. With other ailments, you go to the doctor, they tell you what they are going to do and then fix it. Prostate cancer is not that way. You are going to have to make some very big decisions that can make you feel as though you are very alone. You will need to step back every now and then and take deep breaths. Don't be rushed: take the time you need to feel as good as you can about your decision. Sleep is very important, playing a pivotal role when you are making decisions and recovering from anything, and cancer is no exception. One step at a time, I say.

I have travelled this road. I know its dips and turns and blind spots. I know what it feels like to be startled by such a diagnosis. For sure, everybody who sees you standing there will have something to say about which direction to take or which road to travel. Friends, total strangers in waiting rooms, online chat groups, and even I, another total stranger, will try to offer advice. Listen to everybody and listen to nobody: this is your cancer, and it affects everyone differently, including fellow cancer warriors and survivors.

I do want to say that doctors are the exception. A medical professional shouldn't use the word 'cancer' to send a patient into a panic. If you have a good doctor, he or she will offer reliable advice, helping you to seek second and third opinions if necessary and listening to your concerns about the diagnosis.

As you get used to living with your treatments, and in some cases improving your lifestyle to cope with it, you eventually overcome the feelings of inadequacy, insecurity and paranoia. Let me tell you, however, that is only possible with a willing and understanding partner and family.

In looking at how our lives should be lived during a cancer journey, the following comes to mind: happy home, healthy body, loving relationship with your wife/partner, family and friends.

In my particular case, I know that my wife loves me, cares, and wants to help. Still, the constant loss of ability, drive and functionality takes its toll as the mind is put into turmoil. It gets to the point where discussion and understanding are lost, so much so that physical contact is avoided for fear of disappointment. This leads to frustration, anger, and eventually a feeling of rejection. I ask you – how the hell do you deal with that? How do I communicate the feeling of love, the need for love, and the reassurance of physical contact, retraining the parts that have been dormant for years and that are beginning to reawaken?

My pride and joy, metaphorically speaking, is doing its best to respond now. It's coming back to life, but there is some muscle atrophy, some reluctance to return to its former glory due to inactivity. This is a physical, emotional and psychological problem that can lead to a major disruption in a great relationship. Trying to regain my previous sexual relationship with my wife is my innermost desire, for to fail – in my mind – would have adverse consequences. I have found that even looking at other women in public does not stir any emotions sexually or otherwise, so clearly the issue lies within me. My wife and I touch, we kiss, we hug, etc. Once inside the bedroom, however, it's almost as if we are strangers again. Fortunately, we remain close, because, in our world of continuous adult discussion, we have come to understand that a man is 1-2% penis and 98-99% everything else. Men, think about that the next time you feel you are failing your partner as you walk through your prostate cancer journey. If I wasn't on the cocktail of pills that I am on, clearly we would not be having this discussion and I would be facing a different direction and quality of life. Anyone familiar with cards knows the role luck plays, but that the skill is in the player.

Learning the game is part of playing well, but you only have the cards you have. Sometimes, you just have to work through this hand and hope the next hand is better, as all things go through cycles. You must do what you can with what you have at the time.

I was dealt a bad set of cards to deal with – in medical terminology, advanced metastatic prostate cancer, the worst hand you could be dealt. I did not blame the 'dealer' or the other players in the game for these cards or this diagnosis. I just played the hand the best way I knew how. You may ask why it is important to play the hand you are dealt. Really, what other hand are you going to play? Some get dealt a great hand – early diagnosis, treatment and cure. Others take an average or even poor hand, with a diagnosis of cancer that has escaped the prostate into the bones or lymph nodes and works it into a miraculous winner. However, there are those who will squander even the best hand. Which are you?

Ask yourself what ignites the courage in you to come back again; to keep going, again and again? No matter how many times I got knocked down, I kept getting up, because lying down and giving up was not an option.

I became skilled at the game because my approach to life's adversity was to have a positive attitude and outlook along with realising that each hand would be different as I trod my journey.

This to me is the way you play the hand you are dealt, because sooner or later, your luck will change: it's the law of averages. Remember that it's not just one hand that you will play but many. In my opinion, though, having said all that I have said, cards are not the best analogy for life (after all I was not your avid card player anyway). The wagers are fixed, and for someone to win, the others must lose (in many cases their lives). I don't believe life is a zero-sum game, or the wealthiest people in the history of the world would have been the first ones to call themselves human because we've been subdividing the spoils ever since.

I believe it is both possible, ethical, and practical to help others learn how to play the game better – after all, that's why we have human rights, isn't it? Every human being is entitled to an 'absolute right' to life. We are rarely in direct competition with anyone (or, put differently, there are far more people we do not compete with than those we do compete with).

There is no 'one size fits all' treatment for prostate cancer. All you can do is learn as much as possible about the disease and the many treatment options available and discuss them with your specialist doctor. We are informed that there are more than two hundred different types of cancer, some minor and some less advanced, but in my opinion, there is only one type of cancer: the 'bad' cancer, because each type can cost a life. I was asked once how I held my head up so high after all I've been through. I replied that it's because no matter what, I'm a survivor and not a victim.

17: Why did I not see this coming?

Why did I not see this coming? Why? Cancer is a disease that I am so familiar with – that could kill me – and I turned my back on it and took my eyes off it. Mother, aunt, uncle and cousins perished because of cancer and here I am fighting for my own existence. For a moment let me travel back to the years preceding my family's demise from cancer.

My mother, Hermelita Elizabeth Elvie, was born in 1925. She was a Jamaican national who travelled to the UK in the early 1950s to work for London Transport before meeting my father, Claudius Levi Samuels, an electrician also working for London Transport. Before long two became one and as the years passed two boys, three girls became the production of that unification. Our parents worked hard and loved us without favour.

I recall my father falling ill in the late 1960s, and that was when he was in his early fifties. He watched as his family surrounded him in his hour of need, as doctors tried to unravel the mysterious illness that had struck him down. It was at this stage that I was introduced to the word DEATH.

'Alfred,' my father would say to eleven-year-old me. 'I'm failing in health and you are the oldest child and may have to stand up as a young man and lead the family before too long.'

Having no real understanding or conception of what he meant, I listened, but it all went over my head. Luckily for us, after extensive medical examinations the doctors attributed his condition to a thyroid issue; Dad survived and the family marched on until the mid-1970s, when my mother was diagnosed with breast cancer, culminating in lung cancer. It was an autumn weekend when the family was summoned to the front living room of our home. A place which we attributed with more happy memories than sad, this was the room we were not allowed in except on a Sunday after dinner to listen to the radio and play records and interact as a family or with a guest. The news was broken to us by both our parents. We listened pensively but were stunned at the news... our mother, no, not our dear beloved mother. They had to be mistaken, but they were not and the reality then started to sink in. Confused, hurt and aghast we sat knowing that the front room would never be the same place again in our memory banks. Our mother, she who held the family together, she who loved us, scolded us and advised us, she who went without eating at times so her children would have food... You cannot fathom the despair amongst us as siblings.

From this point forth she was the centre of attention; whatever she wanted or needed she got, the unity of the family became stronger and Dad was rock solid. He lived through the 1970s, then the 1980s came. I was now a young adult making my way in the world, qualified in electronics and data communication engineering. I was offered an overseas post as an electronic technician with a company based in

Jeddah, Saudi Arabia, at the airport terminal. However, the need for me to be close to my mother made me reject the post. Yes! My main reason was that I wanted to be around my mother to assist in whatever way I could as a dutiful son should. I never ever regretted doing so because a few years later, in 1983, she succumbed to her illness. Unbeknown to us, our aunt – my mother's sister – was also dying of cancer and six months after our mother's death she died also.

Now the penny started to drop as it became clear that our family had a hereditary disease issue; it was called 'cancer' and it was to become a great bane of my life. My mother died on 25th March 1983, four days short of my birthday on 29th March, and for me that too became something that took me many, many years to get over. No more celebrations of my birthday, not that I was a party-goer as such. She may have gone but she was not forgotten, having left husband, children and grandchildren along with family elsewhere. She was my mother, my best friend (someone whom you could talk to about anything in life) and she was the woman I respected. I recollect my godmother telling me at the funeral that my mother had confided in her that she regularly spoke with Jesus, being the spiritual person she was, and she had asked him to allow her to live long enough to see her children grow up. I was twenty-two years old and the youngest was sixteen years of age; in my mind, her request was granted.

We gave our mother a grand send-off befitting a royal funeral. She was an avid churchgoer and her faith meant a great deal to her. I recall on one occasion visiting her at the Royal Marsden Hospital in Surrey, whose care she was under, and the chaplain requesting from her a tape of her Christian beliefs and how they impacted on her cancer journey. This was to be used by the hospital to assist other cancer patients going through their journey. Whilst she lived and after she died her taped belief was a comfort for many others as it impacted on their journeys also.

Six months later my aunt in Jamaica died, also of cancer, and it was becoming evidently clearer that all children associated with my mother's side of the family needed to keep an eye on their health, especially cancer, as we were progressing through life. The issue for me was that youth does not cater for remembering to carry out the due diligence with regards to visiting doctors to ensure that I or my siblings did not fall foul of this dreadful disease. Not until I was diagnosed did I really think about or actively make inroads into understanding cancer.

Never could I believe that the impact felt on me and my siblings was to now be felt by me and my family; how cruel can life be? one asks. My mother suffered from cancer for seven years before she died, and the grieving process was felt for possibly as many years afterwards. Now I am going through my own journey – at present, five years. When calculating, it seems that a third of my life has revolved around cancer, both as a sufferer and watching a loved one die from the disease. To have lived and be surrounded by cancer was and is mentally challenging and physically draining: when will it cease? When will I ever get a break? When will my family and friends be able to breathe a sigh of relief?

The pendulum axe of death swings slowly each and every day, restrained at the moment by hope that one day people will no longer have to face this disease. The one thing for sure is that my mother's fight against cancer was not in vain; I too became a warrior like she was. I have fought this disease like she did, and the only difference is I have survived. The scars of loss remain firmly entrenched in my mind.

The family's demise continued with the death of my uncle, my mother's brother. He died in 1988 of prostate cancer and this greatly affected me. Uncle Rowland was not only my uncle but my friend as well; we shared a sense of business acumen. Just before he died he spoke with me from his hospital bed in the USA, where he was undergoing treatment. 'Alfred,' he said. 'I was just walking one day when this searing pain in the base of my spine and lower back took a hold of me.' This was the start of his painful cancer journey which he did not survive.

I suppose inadvertently I had been given all the necessary information in advance on how to deal with what was ahead of me. Not until my journey started did I realise this and now I can impart to all who read this. Life is strange in the way it twists and turns and prepares you for the future way ahead of time; if only we could foresee and understand it. I am perfectly placed to impart the personal feelings and mental anguish undergone over two decades of my lifetime from both sides of the fence.

18: My partner — my caregiver

I t has been a very long, manic and hectic five years since I was first diagnosed. Like everyone else, I have had my ups and downs from a health perspective. In my case, it's advanced metastatic prostate cancer, which is a life-threatening disease. Like some, I have posted some of my woes, lows, and highs on social media groups within the likes of Facebook in a bid to help others.

But this chapter isn't about me. It is about my wife, Grace, my caregiver. My wife is a highly intelligent, quiet and beautiful woman. She greets everyone with a smile and is extremely polite. However, do not mistake her demeanour, for there is under all of this a lioness, protective of her cubs. She is the person that interacts with me on a daily basis, subsequently having to deal with me when I am at my worst. When my confidence is at rock bottom and my frustrations are off the Richter scale. When the false smile that I have painted on for the rest of the world leaves my face, she becomes the unintended target of an abrupt mood swing. I really do try to isolate myself when I feel that moment coming on, but sometimes I fail miserably. When we are supposed to have an entertaining evening out, I am excusably tired. But she is unsure of which type of tired – the 'long day at work tired,' the 'physical exertion tired,' or the 'cancer fatigue tired.'

She is the one left to watch TV by herself because I have gone to bed early. Again! I really wish I could have stayed up a little later, but I was completely exhausted. Again, I meant to ask her about her day – and really listen – but I forgot. Again and again and again it continues. As cancer patients, we become very selfish when our entire focus turns inward in an effort to shut out the rest of the world. We also do this to deny feelings we can't deal with or in an effort to examine why our bodies have betrayed us; tunnel vision then becomes the end result.

At the initial outset, I did not share with my wife my feelings of grief, anxiety and being overwhelmed because I thought it would be adding to the misery. But when I did, I found out that we shared many of the same feelings and it opened my eyes to how deeply she cared for me.

So far on this journey, I have taken pride in the fact that I have not had to give up any of my daily activities. Working, walking or family time, I can and still do them all (well, sort of) but it comes at a bigger cost each time, and requires much more effort and recovery time on my part than it used to. And once again she winds up paying a lot of that cost.

I know I need to make some adjustments on that and I do try; I try my utmost, honest I do. So let me be crystal clear. Grace, I love you with all my heart and cherish our life together. I could not make this journey without you by my side, and I sincerely apologise for those times when I seemed to take it for granted. I am looking forward to our cruise holiday over the forthcoming months.

For a while in my journey, the desire to take the wrong road registered in my head, but in the end, I listened to her advice and took the right road. This ultimately made all the difference not only to my outcome but to our relationship.

I am a realist. I have no vision of changing the entire world by myself, hence the need to listen to the invaluable advice that is given to me. Throughout, she has prepared the right foods and encouraged me to stay in some sort of physical shape as best as I can. Often, she would revert to her scholarly remarks. She would say that I must be both physically and mentally prepared for the road ahead. She would often refer to the concept of 'a sound body and a sound mind'. She would say a strong body would give me confidence, but it would mean nothing without a strong mind. It was her urging that led me to the point where I despised alcohol. Alcohol and strong drugs do not mix; having witnessed it personally, I can attest to that fact.

I no longer wanted anything to do with that which altered my conscious state. I wanted nothing in my body's system that made me less prepared to deal with what was going on around me on a daily basis. Grace was my happiness; being with her brought a smile to my face. I had the best of all worlds in her. She is loving, strong and knowledgeable about the medical world. She has a sincere interest in seeing my mission of remission evolve, not because I am a dad, the head of the family, but because she truly loves me. She sees in me the strength needed to face the task at hand, the strength to stand up to this disease! I would often stare into her eyes and put one arm around her and run my other hand through her hair. I could tell she worried that I might not make it through, as I would often grimace in obvious discomfort from the pain that the cancer was causing.

On many cold winter evenings, we would cuddle up together and kiss and I would whisper into her ear, 'Baby, I'm going to fight and beat this disease, don't you worry now.' I am thankful for the woman I know as my wife, for in times of sickness and dire situations, we have been there for each other. Upon my cancer diagnosis and journey to date, she has kept me going when I wanted to quit and give in.

She has paid attention to every aspect of my physical and mental well-being, often surveying me to ensure I am still physically whole, for she has already taken time out to ensure I am spiritually sound. She always ensures I keep up the fight because she knows that a broken man would mean a broken family and that is not happening whilst she has breath in her body.

We found each other in our later years in life and helped to build each other, and over the years we had become one in the body. Divorce or separation was not in our vocabulary. It was not our way, though there were those who would wish to break down that which was strong and good and see us fall apart. However, our very union was dependent on our ability to see past these façades. There could never be a parting as we would let no one or nothing divide us, not even cancer.

Often I have thought we had missed our vocation as marriage guidance councillors. We have never needed psychologists to sit down with us and work things out. That is not to say ours is a perfect marriage, because it is not. What it is comprised of, though, is definitely honesty, openness, trust, friendship and love. This was more evident during the time when I was hospitalised, when her every visit I yearned for. Around me, as I lay very ill, were those even sicker than I. Some, in fact, were dying and I felt myself slipping into their abyss.

Then my angel would turn up to save me and brighten up my day and so it continued until discharge date. My partner has never portrayed to me the acts of someone 'not being there' for me, nor being basically selfish and delegating duties to others. She has always said that all she wants to do is be there for me. The bottom line is that she is truly an amazing woman!

In retrospect, I tip my hat to all of you who are caregivers. God bless each of you who have set your life apart to take care of the many of us who cannot care for ourselves.

I recall, in the first year of my diagnosis, going from being a very active male with an active partner to almost an invalid, pigeon-stepping male unable to walk short distances and crippled with pain... My wife, who had been an active part of my life before, now had to deal with my emotional transformation to that of a cancer patient. Accepting help from her was extremely hard as I still tried to do things for myself, for I had always been the rock in the family; now I was a mere pebble. As time progressed, though, I was ever so mindful that she could end up with health problems of her own, making it physically and emotionally harder for her to take care of me further.

On reflection, I do believe that she took too much on to herself, although accepting help from others wasn't always easy. We received lots of support, and some of it came from people we expected it from. But a lot came from those we didn't know very well. And others, whom we did know well, stayed away. We wondered on many occasions why some close family members wouldn't offer to help us as they were well aware of what we were dealing with. You just never know with people. So the tendency to just get on with it became the ritual. Through our meaningful conversations, I know we both felt resentment and stress building up within us over the years. But as time progressed, we both learned to just let it go. It wasn't worth the energy expended on it.

Fortunately for me, I have a partner who fully understands my prostate cancer medical situation, as her father had succumbed to the disease. Thus, I always felt confident that she was in control. It was hard on many occasions to find the positives, as we journeyed through, but I constantly thanked my wife for all she has done and continues to do. After all, a simple thank you and thoughtful gesture at times made her see how grateful I am as we continue down the feel-good-factor road. We firmly believe that we have been given the chance to build on and strengthen our relationship as a result. This doesn't mean that caring for me is easy or stress-free. But finding meaning in caring for someone can make it easier to manage.

19: Prostate cancer and the man you love

I have to applaud my wife because, in a way, she suffers the disease too. You might think that prostate cancer sufferers live in a world where life is wonderful and everyone around them is happy and living a normal life, but unless you have walked in their shoes you have no idea. No one knows the real picture. Anyone with the disease suffers financially, emotionally, mentally and physically.

I know exactly what it means to go through all of these. And I apologise to anyone who thinks I'm being too candid – but I can only say it the way I experienced things. The man you have now is a comparative stranger. He is not the man you loved, married, cohabited with, laughed with and had a wonderful intimate relationship with. That man has gone now, maybe never to return. You now have to deal with someone that you now only recognise physically, but not much in any other way. But the love you felt for the 'old him' is still intact and will never go away, and that is why you continue to fight for this 'other him' – the 'new him' – and do everything you can to care for him. The difference now is that you have to do it without any of the little rewards you used to get. The meaningful, passionate kisses, the strong arms entwined around you when you're upset, making you laugh, and the sexual caressing. These are the things you will miss about 'him' so much and that's why I think it's very important to recall appropriate marriage vows: 'for better, for worse; for richer, for poorer; in sickness and in health, until death do us part.'

Sometimes it may feel as if your loved one is already dead (though they are clearly in front of you breathing and ever living) and you think it is the absolute cruellest thing that can happen to a previously happy, loving couple. However, all you can but do at this moment in time is to keep your feelings and words to yourself, in the deepest, locked-away area of your soul. You know, the place where you say things that you dare not admit, but which are true. The tears freely trickle down your face as you cry, not only for your partner and yourself but for all the other wives and partners out there, because you know they feel exactly the same. *God, how I hate this disease. It's so evil and destructive. If only I could have my life back. If only I could have my partner back. If ONLY...*

For me, the interference in my testosterone started the downward roll...The hormone injection Prostap, administered every eight weeks, massively affected my testosterone level. Testosterone is a very powerful hormone. Testosterone is what makes us men, MEN. It is the hormone that gives us larger bones than our female compatriots, heavier muscle mass and bodily hair. It feeds our brains and sex drive. I recollect TV ads that cited the benefits of testosterone replacement therapy! 'Feel young again and have all the energy and sex drive you had as a young man.' For me, it is a sad fact of life that I may never feel that way again, as much as I try. For both of us, it's a thing of the past. It's sad but true. That's just how it is right now. We cannot change the cards we have been dealt; we just have to play the hand we have.

Add the side effects that are real, such as hot flashes, fatigue, depression and loss of sex drive – these are things we face almost daily. But a saviour on a gallant steed came to our rescue in the form of exercise. This has proved to be a saviour and an answer. It has kept my ever-shrinking muscle mass toned. Exercise is not a four letter word. However, there were times during an exercise that I would utter certain expletives in protest at the torturous act I was inflicting on myself. The cursing does not last long, however, for at the end of a session, I realise that my life depends on it more so than at any time in my earlier life.

Treadmills, free weights and hill walking with a weighted rucksack (make your choice) are the selections available to me. Nowadays I do not take my exercise routines to the extreme; a lovely leisurely walk is more than enough. I recall with bitterness the earlier days of my illness where I would observe myself in front of a mirror. In doing so it was evident that all that was left was this fast-fading muscle-bound guy that once was, but no more. Mirrors do not lie; they reflect the soul of the person in front of them. And being upset was a light description of how I felt at what I saw at the time. The greatest benefit now is that I feel good about myself and what is reflected.

As for my sex drive, well, that's another matter altogether for I am not one to venture down the path of the blue pills. I have never used a pill and never will. So I have to give much thought into pleasuring and loving my wife in other, non-sexual ways. If I am actually honest, I get a buzz from doing this now. As men, we tend to focus on ourselves far too much when it comes to affairs of the heart and intimacy. Indeed, most of us are selfish if the truth be told. We think that the world revolves around the size of our penis. Some of us go to extreme lengths to ensure that this is the case, too. But here I am now forced to focus now on something besides my penis. Now my emotions are taking over. In the early, days I used to cry often and it was this that made me really understand what a woman goes through that we take for granted. Now I have learnt to love with my heart. It is a paradigm shift. Focusing my full attention on my wife is the direction I am looking at now.

20: *I have faced fear*

It does not matter where you are from, whether it's the United Kingdom, United States, Europe, Asia, Africa or New Zealand, you cannot escape this tsunami. It has intruded into every corner of the globe; it has engulfed this planet and wreaked havoc on men, women and children alike. It has torn apart husbands, fathers and wives, mothers from their precious children and grandparents from their grandchildren. It is the curse and scourge of our time: the dreaded disease called cancer.

I have faced this fearsome disease, and so many times over the past five years of my journey I have felt that I might not survive. I suppose as normal human beings we all pass through some sort of life experience from time to time in our lives. But right now, for all cancer sufferers, it must be said: what a time to be alive. Never has so much information been at the fingertips of so many of us. In the developed world, technology has made it possible and we are now privileged to have near-instant electronic access to the accumulated knowledge of medicine and how it affects mankind, including up-to-the-minute scientific understanding.

Concurrent with this ready availability of data, we the patients have been encouraged and empowered to advocate for ourselves by searching for cancer content online that is pertinent to our own condition.

However, it is also true that the great guru 'Dr Google' does not supplant the significance and rigour of medical training, so there is real value in enabling dialogue within the healthcare community, both broadly and on an individual scale. This for me means seeking real input and advice from people who have relevant experience and expertise in living with the conditions or situations authors are writing about. We the patients are no longer sitting on the sidelines; we are engaging and becoming an integral part of the research process from beginning to end.

Facebook group chat rooms are plentiful, but the hidden dangers lurk behind as we bear our souls to invisible faces as we find ourselves talking with unqualified but open, honest, eager-to-listen people. Clearly a failing of our NHS system? Yes, I would say without hesitation. It must be said, though, without the internet as a means of immediate and direct information that filters down to the masses on Twitter, Instagram or otherwise, that it would have taken many years for them and their families to have received and digested the research information.

I have found that these days, I do not pay attention to the notion of the world ending because for me it ended when I was diagnosed with cancer. Since then it has ended for me many more times and begun again many more times. I really do not know what happens next, but it's OK. I feel like I'm ready for whatever comes. I'm here and no one really knows what that means except me. I firmly believe that believing we will survive is what makes us survive. When you realise that billions of people in the world are living below the poverty line and surviving on just $2.50 per week, it kind of puts things into perspective: if they can survive, so can I. I have learnt to think of solutions to my dilemma and I do not let my worries control me or stress me out.

I just inhale and exhale, that's how I know everything is all right. I have felt vulnerable whilst opening up my feelings and emotions. My heart and mind have been exposed showing what exists on my inside, clearly bearing too much of myself to those around me – but that's when I realise that I am starting to get it right and that my story can change somebody else's life. Being real is the only way to be. Sometimes the future changes quickly and completely and we are left only with the choice of what to do next. We can choose to be afraid of it, or stand there trembling in fear, not moving, assuming the worst that can happen or we step up into the unknown and assume it will be wonderful.

Maybe it's not supposed to be easy for me – maybe I am one of the rare few who can handle tough times and still choose to be a loving person. Maybe it's going how it's going because I'm built for it. So, therefore, I won't stress myself out about it, it's going to work out because I'm not going to stop putting the work in. Shit happens to people who can handle it. I was made to be this brave human who does not back down to the things in life that try to tidal wave over you and force you to be small. The worst time of my life has turned into the greatest dream of my life, having published not one but two books in relation to prostate cancer. I have been assigned this mountain to show others that it can be moved.

Rest assured that you never believe that the storm is completely over;

you are always wondering, 'will it return and, if so, with what severity?' The most important thing that I've done this year (2017) is to SURVIVE – I have been given a second chance at life and I intend to make everyone proud of me.

I never believed in miracles, but now I do, having undergone stage four advanced metastatic prostate cancer and now showing a regular PSA reading of less than 0.1ng/ml. It's surreal, considering the prognosis five years ago, but now it's time to live my life. My secret to beating cancer is quite simple – keep it going, don't stop.

21: Facing the consequences but marching on

I have entered the fifth year of my advanced metastatic prostate cancer journey, deemed in the medical world as a significant milestone. 'Prostate cancer survival rates have tripled in the UK in the past forty years. Ninety-four percent of men survive prostate cancer for at least one year. This falls to around eighty-five percent surviving for five years or more, which means that most patients can be considered cured after five years. Eighty-four percent of men are predicted to survive their disease for ten years or more.' *(http://info.cancerresearchuk.org/cancerstats/ faqs/#How)*

My goal post-diagnosis was always remission and not merely survival. I have always felt the need to help and assist those recently diagnosed with cancer, and those currently going through the journey. Still, many men are not heeding the call for a better understanding and awareness of this disease, and they are not being tested for the disease at earlier stages of their lives. Though at times I feel intense pain, I walk through those pain barriers for I am that warrior and that voice for those who do not believe they can beat that which seeks to destroy. My previous book, *Invincibility in the Face of Prostate Cancer: Coming Out the Other Side*, opened a new side of me, which was a raw emotional window into me, not only as a person but also as a cancer survivor. I have entered into another phase of a three-phase journey, which includes living with cancer, living through cancer, and living beyond cancer.

At the beginning, when I was first diagnosed, that was the stage of living with cancer. Treatment starts and includes surgery, chemotherapy, and radiation, depending on how far your cancer has progressed. The treatment may accelerate, meaning that surgery may not be an option, and chemo, via IV or orally through tablets, is the first course of action. In my opinion, living with cancer is one of the hardest stages. Consultation with your doctor on a regular basis becomes the norm. At this stage, you are dealing with the physical and emotional demands that living with cancer creates.

The next step is living through cancer. This is the stage after treatment for cancer, better known as the transition stage. It is during this time that many so-called cancer survivors struggle with finding their 'new normal', the new you. Some may feel that their cancer has changed them, their perspective, their personality and their lifestyle. Many are fearful of their cancer returning.

As I sit here pondering the prostate cancer diagnosis I was given five years ago, I cannot help but think about the horrendous impact it had on my life. 'Disabled' and 'retired' are not words that sit well with me. Going from the man who protected physical life to now having to protect his own life from something that there was no medical cure for

– advanced metastatic prostate cancer – is nothing short of jarring. Do I like it? No. Am I going to die? Yes, and so are you: these are the real facts of life. Personally, I think it is time we, as a society, take the strangeness out of the word 'death'. Each day it is becoming less strange to me, and focusing on living rather than dying has helped me to deal with the situation at hand.

The further thought of retirement due to a chronic illness did not bear thinking about. Preoccupied with doctor's appointments, blood tests, MRI and PET scans, the thought and idea of retirement was remote. Most people, including myself, keep on working because we cannot afford to retire, or even worse, we are forced into retirement because of the side effects of treatment.

In some cases, the loss of daily contact with special friends at work felt worse than dying; it was better to hold on to them as long as possible. I am one of those lucky guys who for years have looked forward to going to work each day and on most occasions have achieved this. Now I am alone on my journey and am finding it hard to adjust to my loneliness. The loneliness I refer to is that in my head. This for many has proven to be a deadly combination, myself included. Sitting for hours on end at home, talking with myself, trying to rationalise what was happening and what was going to happen tore at my inner most feelings and mental sanity.

Yes, the moments came where my thoughts drifted toward what the end would be like, how long it might be, and how the time leading up to it would unfold. However, I then realised that it was a defeatist attitude creeping in, and automatically I went back to focusing on living rather than dying.

Complicating the matter was the fact that the medical world had no cure for this disease, nor knew why the disease affects far more black males than Caucasians (one in four opposed to one in eight). With the odds heavily stacked against me and the dice thrown, my life started to unravel in a bid to thwart the disease. From a healthy, fit-for-duty bodyguard to an unfit, sickly individual; my mental anguish was insurmountable as I reflected back on my days of protective duties to the stars.

For near on thirty years of my life, my profession was that of an international bodyguard. During this time, I protected many corporate bodies as well as celebrities in the music and film industries.

I worked with Bob Dylan. He always walked at a fierce pace with minimal conversation between us, which never bothered me. After all, I was there to protect him, not be his friend, and lacking in pace was never apparent from either of us. There would be many other times when we would walk from our hotel to a local recording/rehearsal studio. A particular level of fitness was certainly needed to keep up.

Sade, the queen of cool music, was another artist I protected, and many, including myself, were surprised at her agility and sprint speed – she was an Olympic athlete in the making. At many a show, after her performance she would leave directly off the stage and, without warning, sprint towards the backstage exit to our waiting tour bus. Fortunately, in my younger days, I was a school and athletic clubs sprint champion, and this had carried me into my older age, allowing me to keep up with her and impressing her no end.

Now, none of this mattered at all. I was far removed from the world of music artists and their protection. I was on my own, fighting for my life against a torrid situation. Here and now the usual rules of protection did not apply. What struck me came at me like a thief in the night stealing away my physical and mental ability to function as a man, let alone a human being.

The slowness with which the disease came at me, and then the rapid deterioration thereafter of myself, was to me the most surprising aspect of all. Hot flashes became a daily occurrence. My long, bounding strides were reduced to pigeon steps that even a tiny tot could surpass. I recall a time during my illness when I would go for short walks in my local park. On many occasions I would see this elderly woman walking slowly through a hilly part of the park. She had to be in her eighties. I decided on one occasion to let her have a fifty-yard start on me. This gave me something to aim toward; I would increase the pace of my strides and finally overtake her. I never caught her: it was as if this elderly woman gained a new lease of life. Embarrassed, confused, deflated was how I felt, but I was also sure that my career as a bodyguard was finished. Now, another chapter in my life was about to commence.

I was not ready for it.

22: Three years, now five years – what elation!

From a personal perspective and forward thinking at the time of diagnosis, I have reached the second of two milestones that I set myself. I surpassed three years in 2015, now in 2017 I have reached my fifth year since diagnosis for advanced metastatic prostate cancer. Who said I no longer had it in me? Let me tell you, you do keep fighting. What I had prayed for, yearned for was now indeed a reality. If I had listened to what my GP had said about my chances, I would have put myself into the ground well ahead of my appointed time. I kept strong to the hope that lay within as I struggled to overcome. The reason why this was happening they didn't know, which complicated matters in my mind further. I won't delve further into the intricacies of the modern medical world as to cures or remissions. I am happy and thankful for the things that have been done and the things that are being done in the name of cancer research.

My heart is trying to scream out for joy, but my tongue is tied, so a muted response is all that I can try. Everyone now assumes the war is won and thinks that I am cured, when in fact it's only just started. I was always in it for the long haul; shame most of you were not. Most of you have gone home because you think the war is won.

A few have stayed, not realising I now need you closer than ever to see it out. My wife is a great medical advocate; she is my ray of sunshine acting as a beacon helping me to navigate through the troubled waters. Ours is a relationship unlike anything I have experienced before in my life. She has been supportive in every step that I have made: every doubt, fear, anxiety, and triumph. Ours is a relationship that many are envious of, without which I would not have made it through, and for that reason I have the greatest admiration for her.

These five years have meant so much to her and her face shows the bubbly joyful mood she is in. The champagne is on chill as the weekend approaches and I know I will partake in it if only a glass in appreciation of all she has done. Even to this day, I am unable to put it all behind me. Frightened, apprehensive, depressed and sad are just a few of the feelings I experience when I think about the future and attempt to plan anything with my wife. It has been extremely difficult living with my cancer and the notion that it may come back is a haunting possibility. Even my oncology team cannot be certain that my cancer has gone for good, and for me, it's very upsetting that no one can say for sure 'Yes, you are cured.'

This is why a cancer diagnosis is a total life-changer: life is never the same again. As you progress through this dark murky journey as I have done, there comes a point in time when you realise that nothing will ever be the same, and you realise that from now on, time will be divided into two parts: before this shit happened and after this shit happened. For me, these five years have hung around my neck like an albatross. I thought a smile would come back to my face, along with boundless amounts of energy to my body but this has not been the case.

Do I feel elated? Do I feel mentally free? Hell no! Not at all. I recently lost a friend to the disease, so celebrations are not something at the top of my list, but that's not to say my family is not thinking about it. I have sensed as I have edged towards this five-year-mark that the feeling of elation would not be all that. I had imagined the sky full of rainbows, different coloured balloons floating in the air, a fanfare, medals of some sort being pinned on my chest... All this I see in my headspace, but nothing like that happened – it just felt like another day of another week of another month in my life. In the grander scheme of things, it has been amazing to see how far I have come from a six-month death sentence.

My fifty-ninth birthday is just two months away, and though I won't celebrate it, I'm appreciative of making it to the age. Maybe I'll make sixty, and have something really to celebrate about, but it certainly won't be for these past hard, long, slogged-out years of undergoing treatment for this wretched disease. My days are ruled by side effects, the severity of which varies. Whilst these side effects do not ease up, you do realise that they are there to stay. They never lied to me; they just stretched the truth about the cancer journey. I am a man with a pen and vocabularies to match and never too afraid to voice my opinions in an openly honest manner in a bid to help others and ease through this quagmire of information and at times misinformation in relation to cancer.

I hope your matrimonial situation is similar to mine and you are not going through a cancer journey alone. I truly hope that you are surrounded with love and loved ones as you battle this illness. If as a man you are reading this in support of a father, brother, uncle, or as a woman as a partner or wife, and you feel something is wrong within yourself or not quite right I urge, in fact, I implore you to go to a GP for professional advice. Don't be frightened; think of it as saving your life.

I wonder how many people understand the beauty of visiting an oncology department of a cancer treatment centre, seeing painful expressions on people's faces, but also seeing joyful expressions. Who would have thought pain and joy could coincide in the most extraordinary places; a cancer treatment centre is no exception. I say all of this because I have seen many moments of elation during my journey, maybe enough to last me for a lifetime. Pain and joy split people's lives and it is in these environments that these moments can be clearly seen: grief, darkness, frustration, panic and moments of wonder. I am amazed sometimes how people still look physically wonderful, their dignity not altered by this horrendous diagnosis, that's not to say internally or mentally they are feeling the same, a place I have found myself in so often during this journey. I suppose, in fact, I know that each appointment for me has already been a moment of uncelebrated elation until now. The important five-year marker that I have waited for and worked so hard for arrives, and I ask: so what makes this so different to everything I have witnessed and undergone? Maybe the elation build-up has just worn off, and now I just feel happy and fortunate to be alive.

So to me, life-expectancy charts are useless for the average man, simply because they throw everyone into the same soup pot and spit out a number without factoring in individuals' general all-round health (i.e. high blood pressure, diabetes, obesity, spending fourteen hours a day watching TV while eating cholesterol-rich foods... For some, their idea of exercise is popping the lid on a beer can).

If all or part of the aforementioned applies to you, then you have a problem; if not, then like me, laugh off all the life-expectancy charts. Diet and exercise with a dash of medication that gets pumped into you by your oncology team – love them or hate them, that's what they are there to do. When it comes down to some good old rest and relaxation time, don't put off planning holidays. Enjoy your life; you are not going anywhere for a long, long time. As the years have passed, I have come to realise that I know more about prostate cancer than most oncologists. Let me put it this way, anyone can research, including you. The difference is you are just researching prostate cancer not twenty different cancers like many oncologists out there. So get ready, set, and go. If you have just been diagnosed or know someone who has, then buckle up and get ready for the long ride. That means lifestyle changes and long walks every day to mention but two. Remember most of all, though, to still enjoy your life and stay away from stress – ditch it or hit it for six. Keep away from those blood-sucking vampires that wander this planet with the sole intention of making your life unbearable.

According to my chart reading, I should be dead already. I can tell you one thing for sure, though – the internet is not only awash with stories of people beating the disease, but also with those who have had their condition managed well for example since 1998, 2000, 2012 and so on. It's all about first and foremost taking an active role in educating yourself to banish those helpless feelings into oblivion and get on with living. Obviously I am very appreciative of this good fortune, for it has influenced my thinking and outlook on life. Cancer exposed me to the uncertainties of life and as such, I have learned to put aside my fears, apprehension, and concerns about tomorrow and appreciate what I have now. I still believe – I must believe – that at some stage a procedure or pharmacologic agent will rid me of this disease and restore life and, hopefully, quality of life as I experienced prior to my diagnosis. The future is bright with a wealth of developing treatment possibilities on the horizon. Maybe just maybe, I will have something to be really elated about after all.

23: Cancer: a struggle, a battle and a fight

Many people think of the words 'struggle', 'battle' and 'fight' when the topic of cancer comes up in a conversation. If you were to take the definition of these words literally, you would probably think of a wartime situation. But it is appropriate to use these words when talking about cancer because to those suffering from cancer it can feel like a struggle, battle and fight every single day. They actually like hearing those words because it gives them a feeling of positivism and accomplishment. This is especially true when a cancer patient has been diagnosed with stage four cancer, which refers to advanced metastatic prostate cancer.

You might think a cancer patient is basically waging war on themselves when they use these words, but it is simply the mindset they need to have to keep their sanity. That is why I do not feel bad about using these words because they have assisted me in my journey thus far.

As someone with advanced metastatic cancer, I struggle, battle and fight against it every day so I can stay alive and be there for my family. This is just one reason, though. I also fight this cancer to honour all those who have died from it or been diagnosed with it. And lastly, I fight this cancer to honour those people who will eventually also be diagnosed with cancer.

The closest people in my life have been there to support me. When they look into my eyes, they see only a fraction of the pain I feel as I continue moving forward on the bumpy road of life. On top of that, I continue to deal with the side effects of the medications that I must take, medications that hurt me at the core of my mental and physical well-being.

There are moments when I feel I can control my symptoms, while at others it feels like cancer is overpowering me. Even though I have no sexual function and feel extremely fragile, I do my best to function like a human being. This can be extremely difficult when you're suffering from cancer. However, I have found that meditation is the key to improving my mental health. I have learned to accept that cancer chose me and I didn't choose it, so I must learn to live with the situation and make the best of it.

It is tough, though, because cancer does not care about your body, soul or mind. It will destroy whatever it wants to destroy. The worst part is that the tumours growing in the body have cancer cells that tend to break away and move through the bloodstream to other areas of the body. Once these cancer cells get there, they cause new tumours to form in these other locations. That is why I still worry about what will happen to me in the end because there is just so much uncertainty.

No one will ever know my anguish and pain until they have been diagnosed with cancer and endured the same anguish and pain that I have. Only then will they understand the significance behind my silent tears. Only at that point would you be able to say you're sorry for having doubts about what I was experiencing. Perhaps you'll even apologise for believing that I and those like me do not have any feelings.

Sometimes I feel like this cancer has long tentacles that are slowly moving their way throughout my body and grabbing hold of my internal organs in order to kill me.

Let me be a bit introspective about a couple of things: Why does a disease like cancer exist in the first place? Why do people have to endure such a degrading disease as this?

I ask myself all the time why nature created this disease. Throughout my life, I have seen how destructive cancer can be. I am a son, nephew, uncle, husband and father, so I am not about to give up just yet, because I have a great deal to live for. Now that I am facing my fifth year of cancer, the idea of there being a cure is something that I am hopeful for. I'm more open to trying out any kind of treatment, whether it's conventional, alternative or natural. I have already used numerous treatment products and I am amazed how helpful they have been throughout this process for me. Although I am realistic about the fact that there's little chance of finding a cure, I am confident that there's a treatment out there which will help make my cancer more manageable for me and for those like me.

Cancer is a term that the media has thrown around a lot. However, it is still such a complicated disease that people tend to just label it. Cancer is not about labels and I do not subscribe to these labels. All I try to do is live my life the best way I can. I elected to make a choice between life and giving up; I chose life. I'm trying to keep a positive outlook toward the future and I will be taking positive actions towards preserving my life.

24: Always hope – there's still life to live

I t's a sad fact that we go through much of our lives on autopilot, not really engaging at all with the things around us. We work hard, sure, and we try to do a good job, but then we come home and we're tired and we just want to have some dinner, watch some TV and go to bed early enough to have the energy and zest to do it all again the next day. And so life revolves.

Well, cancer has a little something to say about that. When you're diagnosed with cancer – even one of the so-called 'good' cancers – the first thing you see is the existential threat. I suppose it must be related to the 'fight or flight' response. We receive the diagnosis. We see the threat. We know that the rest of our life might be measured in months and weeks instead of years. We're very afraid indeed; in fact, we are petrified. It's perfectly natural. Most people are afraid of death or, if not of death, then of dying, because they're two separate things. But after a little while, you realise something. Everyone's going to die. We all know this, but we don't all understand it. You're going to die. I'm going to die. The youngster at the coffee shop who doesn't look old enough to drive, who sold you your morning coffee, is going to die. The little kids playing at the park are going to die—a long time from now, we hope, but it's going to happen.

Once you have this realisation, that dying is part of living, you have the realisation that living is part of dying. Because when your days are numbered, you should really want to make them count.

At some level, I think we're all trying to live a life worth living. When you receive that diagnosis, your standards for what is worth living get a damn lot higher and – spoiler alert – spending more time at work doesn't really count for anything anymore.

You want to spend more time with your family. You want to spend more time with your friends. You want to spend more time doing things that really matter.

Because let's face it, a lot of the things we do in life don't really matter. What matters is being a good husband or wife. What matters is being a good parent. What matters is being a good friend. What matters is not increasing productivity, what matters now is living life, seeing the world, and hopefully leaving it just a little better than you found it. I am a prostate cancer survivor. I have lived through the side effects and nausea and everything. I have lived through the fear, I have lived through the pain, the doubt and mostly everything else associated with this disease.

When life hands you a cancer diagnosis, there are only two options. You can roll over and take it, or you can realise that you're invincible. For a long while in my life, I walked with a certain cockiness of invincibility and as such approached everything I did in the same manner, but I suppose to a certain extent that's a male for you. To accept the fact that my body armour of invincibility had betrayed me and allowed this disease to penetrate was unacceptable. Here I was, this hard-working male who regularly worked 18-hour days, sometimes longer. My perspective on life was now challenged; what had been under control for so long was dishevelled and uprooted and I was faced with starting all over again and I was far from ready for such a situation.

But time was not on my side and the need to reorganise myself and my family quickly presented itself on my doorstep. With head held high, I slowly commenced the restructure of my life and gradually realised that there was hope after all and I was still alive and still able-bodied. The resurrection of my life was well under way, but with a twist. Prostate cancer was now a new part of me because no matter how many times this illness knocked me down, I had conditioned myself that giving up was not an option, and neither was lying down. You see, a regular daily Q&A session was undergone as I found the courage to ignite, coming back again and again from each blip that kept me going on, again and again.

I knew I had the courage because I looked deep into myself at every opportunity. The side effects of my medication at times made life seem unbearable, but I can think of far worse things that can make life intolerable. I'll just stick with the side effects in the hope that one day a cure will be found to end this life-limiting journey.

25: Afraid to say, won't say, saying the wrong things

How I wish people would truly understand the psychology of a person who has just been diagnosed with cancer. This life-threatening disease poses a different set of circumstances that makes understanding it a fairy tale. It's very difficult to judge the well-being and emotions of someone just by perusing his or her outward countenance. Most of the time healthy people may not know how to empathise with them. I keep hearing comments about how great I look, even with my diagnosis of stage four advanced metastatic prostate cancer.

I am still considered by many as one and the same as before my illness, but subsequently the phone calls begin to drop till I eventually stop hearing from them. The cancer disease has made me different because I feel my life ebbing away slowly.

I have heard comments from people along the lines of 'You are so brave, I don't know if I could do it'. Honestly speaking, the fight against cancer makes us heroes because we battle a disease that scares the hell out of a lot of people. Our strength comes from our inner desire to live and our refusal to succumb to this sickness, hence we face all sorts of diagnoses, therapies and side-effects that are more painful than the ailment itself.

We show courage because even when we find it difficult listening to the heartbreaking lab results, we are left with no choice but to take in whatever devastating news the tests bring.

Living with cancer

The reality of living with cancer is far removed from the picture portrayed. The battle is simply choosing living over dying, even when the odds are against you, because, other than that, death seems to be the only option.

Strength: We adapt to the pain and the illness as a second chance at life.

Braveness: We develop the attitude of coping and accepting the things we cannot change.

Faith: Belief in God handles the questions we can't answer.

The reality of being a cancer patient is rarely about the challenges one is facing, because they do all it takes to be brave, to try and make people around them understand what they are going through each minute of each hour of each day. Time has no limit or end.

Let's be clear and hit the nail on the head; I and other cancer patients don't have the luxury of time.

Cancer: Ten things to note (in all honesty)

1. Don't expect me to call you if I am in need

I would love it if you called me occasionally and scheduled a visit to see me. Yes, you have told me several times to call you if I am ever in need, but I am uncomfortable with putting up with such calls before we get to spend time together or before you help me to do things I once used to do efficiently. I hate the feeling of dependency, and I get scared you'll give me tiresome excuses.

2. I need to be emotional at times

I agree with you that cancer and its treatment are taking a toll on me and this affects my personality. But I don't want to be shut out of showing empathy in certain circumstances. I am still a normal person with emotions and feelings and when I am angry please understand and know that someone or something has annoyed me. Don't brush it off as an effect of cancer. Please afford me the liberty to express myself when and how I want to, as I did before the illness.

3. I prefer 'Hey, what's up?' to hearing 'How do you feel?' all the time

I would prefer we talk about politics, life, religion, governance or anything that interests me than always speaking of cancer. It's depressing, trust me.

4. Be forgiving

At times the sickness and treatment make me lose touch with myself. Whatever trait I portray at such times that hurts, annoys or irritates you, it was never done intentionally. Try to forgive me at these moments in time; I have changed from the person you used to know.

5. Listen to me

It takes every fibre of my being to be strong. When it seems like I am down and depressed, all I need from you is a listening ear. In such times allow the tears to flow as it eases the pain and gives me a measure of peace and inner strength.

6. Take pictures of us together

I know you sometimes wonder why I insist on having photographs all the time. Photographs strengthen me during depressing times, and they are a way of remembering what a treasure I am. I hate saying 'don't remember me this way' when chemotherapy and all the therapy science has to offer leaves me bald and looking funny. Appreciate me now; that person you see before you now is what I want you to remember.

7. I want to be alone

In the beginning, I talked about how I needed you to spend time with me. Well, now all of a sudden I need to be alone. I will always love you and cherish our times together, but sometimes I need the detachment of laying down the mask of bravery, behind which faded dreams, hopelessness and sadness exist.

8. My family needs friends

It's difficult when you are living a normal life to deal with the day-to-day running around. Imagine how much more difficult it becomes dealing with all that stuff with a cancer diagnosis or treatment on the other hand. My wife needs friends to spend time with her, not necessarily to replace my vacuum but to ease the stress and do things I would have ordinarily loved to do with her. I feel happy knowing you also care about my family.

9. I also want you to reduce your risk of cancer

I would hate for anyone to face this. I agree that you cannot avoid some cancers. However, you can reduce your risk of having cancer with an adjustment to how you live – don't smoke, maintain a regular weight, avoid excessive exposure to sunlight and eat healthy foods. It's necessary you keep regular appointments with the doctor and don't hesitate to follow up such appointments when worrisome symptoms emerge. A lot of people still have a fair chance at life if cancer is discovered early. It's my desire that you live a healthy life.

10. Take nothing for granted

Live your life to the fullest. Take time out to have a series of adventures while appreciating God for nature and the existence of man.

It may be difficult to see the good in cancer or be thankful for it, but we should not fail to realise the help that medical science has offered, and the aid that comes to fight this deadly disease via treatments, and for that we should be grateful. If such a time comes, when my body builds resistance to the treatments and therapies, never forget that I will always appreciate God first and foremost, and my life spent with you and the family we have built.

There is only one woman I have ever loved this past five years. She is my treasured love, a wonderful woman indeed. We have shared our lives, memories, laughter, tears, sadness, and pains together.

Also, know this: I don't want you ever to pity me. My continued existence is a miracle. My oncology team is of this view, and I kick against it. All I desire is to be who God wants me to be, whether I am sick or strong, and when I defeat cancer all I want to hear from you is 'You are the hero'.

Some hate it when others desire to pray for them. I was happy when people offered to pray for me. In 2012 my GP told me I would not live beyond six months and a year at most and yet I am still breathing. Prayers are effective for me and when you have the attitude of praying, miracles are sure to abound – I know that.

Finally, if you hear of someone diagnosed with cancer, send an email, call or write a letter simply to send your sympathy. Ignoring such a message with an intention to make excuses that you did not know what to say is not the decent thing to do.

26: *The new me*

Cancer is a bomb that disrupts your life, causing in my case an enormous, indescribable amount of pain that threatened to take away my identity and turn me into someone else entirely: a cancer patient. Clearly, the person I was yesterday is not the person I am today. I am an ambassador for Cancer Research UK and Go Dad Run – two prominent cancer awareness and fundraising organisations in the UK – and a mentor for Young Enterprise and Urban Synergy, two organisations that help young men and women achieve their goals in life. And the list goes on and on. Would I have ever accomplished any of these positions if I had not been diagnosed with cancer? Probably not, if I am to be honest.

It's incredible: until I wrote my first book *Invincibility in the Face of Prostate Cancer: Coming out the Other Side*, I never guessed that it would have such an emotional effect on its readers. I have received accolades and many good reviews, especially from fellow cancer survivors, who have told me that I was on the right track because I had touched a chord with their own cancer journeys. Clearly, my brothers-in-arms, along with their loved ones, had felt the impact of my sentiments. What was clear, however, was their inability to convey these feelings to those around them, because the subject matter was far from easy to discuss.

What makes this disease such that only a few can relate and discuss in-depth emotional feelings in respect of their own very personal and intimate journeys? We men are hardened so much in life that the affairs of a very personal and sensitive or sexual nature find us cowering in the nearest corner of a room for sanctuary. If only we could be so brave and face our demon cancer, our struggle would be far easier. It's not easy: it's hard changing your life as you try to smooth the rough edges. The cards that life dealt me have changed my perspective in a major way and I love every minute of it. I look deep inside myself now and realise that I have found the 'new me' and everyone loves this new me.

Who was I before this change of circumstances affected my life so drastically? Someone totally unfulfilled, a sad reflection of the old me but at least it's a positive change. I stand tall, upright and pristine like a soldier guarding Buckingham Palace. I talk with wisdom and knowledge on the subject matter of prostate cancer like a university professor, on a disease that I have become ever so familiar with. With this new-found knowledge I am able to apply a strange life-encouraging twist, which encourages not only the youth of tomorrow but also adolescents to listen keenly to my words of wisdom. There were moments when I doubted myself, but I got through because I looked to God to bring me through.

On many occasions I have been asked if I believe in God, primarily because I have never said much about anything when it comes to God. I don't always understand Him, but I believe in God. I don't know what religion he would sanction or disavow, but I do believe in God.

I don't run around with religious pendants on my chest or Bibles and other holy books under my arm. I don't wake people up by knocking on their doors and pushing magazines in their face. I don't stand on the street corner selling newspapers. I surely am not kissing a man's fingers, hand, ring, or any other part of him. I don't chant, but I quietly believe. I can only explain it as something inside me. I believe in 'Know you not that you are the temple of God,' (1 Corinthians 3:16). My church and sanctuary are all inside my soul. I get dressed up and walk through the aisles of my soul and bow to God and pray. I pray for knowledge and understanding. I pray for the daily strength to do what is right and necessary. I'm a stronger believer than many professors of faith.

As I look at myself each day in the mirror, I say: it's not over until I win. No matter what life throws at me today or tomorrow, it can't be any worse than what I have been through already. It's a liberating feeling to know that the words I have written have mattered to so many people. Imagine if I had given up initially upon diagnosis. I never gave up, and here I am today, five years later, looking forward to another five years or more of life. It was a daunting moment when I looked at the challenge ahead, but one step at a time, and with a little rest along the way, I achieved what I thought was impossible.

In this book, *Motivated to Inspire*, I introduce my perspective as a cancer survivor; I introduce my new self to the rest of the world. For me, health anxieties are now a compartment of my new life. It's weird for me to sit here and continue to write and think of myself as a cancer survivor. Ultimately, I am seeking to achieve the elusive 'mission remission,' something rarely heard of in someone with my condition.

I can say two things with equal certainty: the first is that I cannot remember with any real clarity what it feels like not to worry, sometimes obsessively, about my health; the second is that acknowledging this fact causes me great shame. How did I let this happen, having witnessed my own mother's demise from cancer and that of other members of my family? I can only chastise myself for such self-indulgent introspection.

I have witnessed and experienced much loss during these years of sickness. I have listened in horror and sympathy to stories of strong, capable men battling against prostate cancer, losing their hair, remaining strong for partners and children, and just a few emerging triumphant.

Cancer is a disease that I have feared for most of my life, as a result of my mother and other family members succumbing to it. My first fears began to condense into certainties, no less fearful upon receipt of my diagnosis. Due to many anxious moments, I did not feel compelled at first to research my disease for many months.

As my body started to respond to my medication, I then found myself walking a tightrope between happiness and unhappiness. Having cancer does not preclude me from offering a different sense of perspective on life and ways to achieve all that you seek from it. I am often amazed at my ability to impart what I have gone through in such a way that it does not seem morbid, insensitive or boring to my listeners. With every pen stroke, I feel that I am being guided in getting across my points of view. Stagnant I have most definitely not become as the years flow by. This new energy that I find myself possessing is pushing me beyond boundaries that I am able to fulfil. For many, as they approach the age of 60 slowing down is compulsory, but not for me as I find the boundless energy to trudge my way through the daily mire. My mindset says, 'Do what you can do now because tomorrow you are not assured of, so give as much of yourself that you can to those who want and need someone like me in their lives.' Everything I do is voluntary and I ask for nothing in return other than your time to listen to what I am saying. Within me, a sense of accomplishment is achieved when I see people of all ages and creeds acknowledging and grasping the information I impart. To empower and bring out the best in people is not an easy task, but through my writing and old and new experiences, I am able to do so.

I have found that now, more than ever, as I search for reassurance, I want so much to be around to see my grandchildren grow up. This new me now prays regularly – extra politely for maximum effect – that the Almighty keeps my wife, children, and grandchildren safe. I say: 'Dear God, you and I have spoken on many occasions, but recently we have done so more frequently. Please keep all my family safe.' I am not overly religious, and I am certainly not deluded enough to think that God will save me from this disease. What I want, though, is a defence against uncertainty. I want not to die early or to become an incapacitated shadow of my former self, a burden on my wife and my children.

Symptoms such as throbbing headaches and tingling fingers and toes are just some of the side effects to deal with at times. Sometimes I have wondered if this was my mind taking my body into a fearful 'fight or flight' state. However, in the grand scheme of things, the new me was still able-bodied and mentally alert. I am now so hyper-aware of my body that certain sensations felt are at times blown out of all proportion and become part of a spiral of unwanted panic.

Health, they say, is now the second most popular internet search topic after pornography. Millions of people type symptoms and diseases into search engines and wait for some dreadful outcome. The reality is that we terrify ourselves as we read information that we do not understand but use to justify our worst fears. From a personal perspective, the role of the GP seems to be somewhat redundant. As one told me recently, 'People don't trust their GPs anymore. We haven't the time to give patients what they need, and it's resulted in a breakdown of trust. They go on the internet themselves.' Wow! It's so true.

As each year passes, I notch up a further milestone in cancer history and this places me in a unique position that many do not reach. I am that Pathfinder. I know God has a helping hand in the path that I am taking; I feel His ever-present direction in my every move. My relationship with the Father is bringing me closer to fully submitting my life to doing His work, wanting no recompense in return. My recompense is my life, extended life that I have been given so that I may help others be guided towards the light of knowledge and direction.

We have all heard those that have experienced a close-to-death experience say how it changed their lives. However, think about those that experience the same scenario on a more regular basis. I'm not saying that I am infallible or of a Godlike status, far from it. The experience of what I undergo makes me respect life and all those that live it. Some foolishly waste this precious gift that is handed down, and my reasoning for this is that we are not assured what the afterlife brings. You're either part of the problem in life or part of the solution; I would like to think I am the latter. When you make a difference in the daily lives of people who are suffering just like I am, it is wondrous to hear them say that you make the difference to their day in what you say or do.

When I was 12, my mother gave me a small Bible for my birthday, something that I never really appreciated at that time in my life. I remember her words very clearly, as if it were yesterday. When she handed me this gift-wrapped item, she said, 'Son, I can't afford the toys and fashionable clothes that you would have preferred.' Upon opening my gift, a Bible fell into my hands, and inscribed on the inside cover were the following words: 'To my son, Alfred, may this be a guide throughout your life. Love Mum.'

As I face what I face today, I now know the true value of that birthday present. It was the best and most precious present that I have ever received and even now, all these years, later a tear comes to my eye.

Don't lose hope:
when the sun goes down, the stars come out.